CW01263750

NUCLEIC ACID THERAPEUTICS IN CANCER

CANCER DRUG DISCOVERY AND DEVELOPMENT

BEVERLY A. TEICHER, SERIES EDITOR

NUCLEIC ACID
THERAPEUTICS IN CANCER

Edited by

ALAN M. GEWIRTZ, MD

Department of Internal Medicine,
University of Pennsylvania School of Medicine,
Philadelphia, PA

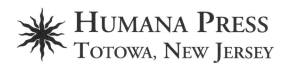

HUMANA PRESS
TOTOWA, NEW JERSEY

This publication is printed on acid-free paper. ∞
ANSI Z39.48-1984 (American National Standards Institute) Permanence of Paper for Printed Library Materials.

Production Editor: Mark J. Breaugh.

Cover design by Patricia F. Cleary.

Cover Illustration: Foreground: Fluorescence microscopy micrographs of HeLa cells incubated with fluorochrome-labeled tat peptides. See Fig. 1, p. 124. Background: Molecular portrait of the reverted phenotype (flat) of PC3M cells and tumors treated with antisense RIα. See Fig. 1, p. 206.

For additional copies, pricing for bulk purchases, and/or information about other Humana titles, contact Humana at the above address or at any of the following numbers: Tel.: 973-256-1699; Fax: 973-256-8341; E-mail: humana@humanapr.com or visit our website at www.humanapress.com

Photocopy Authorization Policy:
Authorization to photocopy items for internal or personal use, or the internal or personal use of specific clients, is granted by Humana Press Inc., provided that the base fee of US $25.00 per copy is paid directly to the Copyright Clearance Center at 222 Rosewood Drive, Danvers, MA 01923. For those organizations that have been granted a photocopy license from the CCC, a separate system of payment has been arranged and is acceptable to Humana Press Inc. The fee code for users of the Transactional Reporting Service is: [1-58829-258-4/04 $25.00] .

Printed in the United States of America. 10 9 8 7 6 5 4 3 2 1

E-ISBN: 1-59259-777-7

Library of Congress Cataloging-in-Publication Data

Nucleic acid therapeutics in cancer / edited by Alan M. Gewirtz.
     p. ; cm. -- (Cancer drug discovery and development)
Papers from a conference held Apr. 2000 in Bryn Mawr, Pa.
Includes bibliographical references and index.
   ISBN 1-58829-258-4 (alk. paper)
 1. Antisense nucleic acids--Therapeutic use. 2. Cancer--Chemotherapy.

 [DNLM: 1. Neoplasms--therapy--Congresses. 2. Gene
Therapy--methods--Congresses. 3. Nucleic Acids--therapeutic
use--Congresses. QZ 267 N9638 2004] I. Gewirtz, A. M. (Alan M.) II.
Series.
  RC271.A69N83 2004
  616.99'4061--dc22
                              2003025020

PREFACE

There is no impossibility that cannot be overcome.
—From *Fateless* by **Imre Kertesz**, Nobel Laureate in Literature, 2002

The development of simple, reliable tools for modifying gene expression "on demand" has stoked the fires of the revolutionary advances being made, on almost a daily basis, in cell and molecular biology. Similar advances are being made in understanding the molecular pathogenesis of many diseases that effect humankind. Not surprisingly, the wish to exploit these advances for the treatment of disease has grown in parallel.

My interest in molecular medicines led me into the field of nucleic acid therapeutics some 15 years ago. Like any developing science, it has had its highs and lows but overall, the movement has been inexorably in a positive direction. In order to spur such progress on, I applied to the Leukemia and Lymphoma Society of America for funds to sponsor a small, and highly focused workshop on basic aspects related to the development of RNA-targeted therapeutics. Monies to supplement the meeting were provided by the Doris Duke Charitable Foundation and the Cancer Center at the University of Pennsylvania. This volume, *Nucleic Acid Therapeutics in Cancer*, largely results from that meeting, which was held in April of 2000 in Bryn Mawr, Pennsylvania.

This volume is small, as was the meeting, but all of the important issues, at least as I view them, are covered in a succinct and highly readable form. These include chapters on RNA biology and the underpinnings of what we now know as RNA interference, oligodeoxynucleotide delivery into cells, strategies for targeting these molecules to accessible regions with the mRNA, and some examples of how these compounds are being used clinically. As such, the collected works should be of use to those who would like an introduction to this field, and present state of the art.

It is my sincere belief that development of effectively targeted, and efficiently delivered, nucleic acid molecules will lead to important advances in the diagnosis and treatment of human malignancies. As was true for the field of monoclonal antibody-based therapies, where hype was followed by disappointment and then finally genuine triumph of the concept, I believe that breakthroughs in the area of nucleic acid-mediated gene silencing will shortly be forthcoming and will more than justify the time and resources expended in developing the therapeutic use of these molecules.

Alan M. Gewirtz, MD

CONTENTS

CONTRIBUTORS

SUSAN J. BASERGA, MD, PhD • *Departments of Molecular Biophysics and Biochemistry, and Therapeutic Radiology and Genetics, Yale School of Medicine, New Haven, CT*

JEAN-PAUL BEHR, PhD • *Laboratoire de Chimie Génétique Associé CNRS, Faculte de Pharmacie, Université Louis Pasteur de Strasbourg, Illkirch, France*

PASCALE BELGUISE, PhD • *Laboratoire de Chimie Génétique Associé CNRS, Faculte de Pharmacie, Université Louis Pasteur de Strasbourg, Illkirch, France*

LUBA BENIMETSKAYA, PhD • *Department of Medicine, Albert Einstein College of Medicine, Bronx, NY*

GORDON G. CARMICHAEL, PhD • *Department of Genetics and Developmental Biology, University of Connecticut Health Center, Farmington, CT*

YOON S. CHO-CHUNG, MD, PhD • *Cellular Biochemistry Section, National Cancer Institute, Bethesda, MD*

NATHALIE DIAS, PhD • *American Language Program, College of Physicians and Surgeons, Columbia University, New York, NY*

DAVID A. DUNBAR, PhD • *Science Department, Cabrini College, Radnor, PA*

FRITZ ECKSTEIN, PhD • *Max-Planck-Institute for Experimental Medicine, Göttingen, Germany*

PATRICK ERBACHER, PhD • *Laboratoire de Chimie Génétique Associé CNRS, Faculte de Pharmacie, Université Louis Pasteur de Strasbourg, Illkirch, France*

ALAN M. GEWIRTZ, MD • *Department of Internal Medicine, University of Pennsylvania School of Medicine, Philadelphia PA*

LIDA K. GIFFORD, PhD • *Department of Chemistry, University of Pennsylvania, Philadelphia PA*

PETER M. GLAZER, MD, PhD • *Departments of Therapeutic Radiology and Genetics, Yale University School of Medicine, New Haven, CT*

JAN S. JEPSEN, BS • *Danish Cancer Society, Copenhagen, Denmark*

R. L. JULIANO, PhD • *Department of Pharmacology, School of Medicine, University of North Carolina, Chapel Hill, NC*

ROSEL KRETSCHMER-KAZEMI FAR, PhD • *Institute for Molecular Medicine, University of Lübeck, Lübeck, Germany*

JOHNATHAN C. H. LAI, BS • *Department of Biomedical Engineering, College of Physicians and Surgeons, Columbia University, New York, NY*

BERNARD LEBLEU, PhD • *UMR5124 CNRS, Institut de Genetique Moleculaire, Universite de Montpellier II, Montpellier, France*

PONZY LU, PhD • *Department of Chemistry, University of Pennsylvania, Philadelphia PA*

JOANNA B. OPALINSKA, MD • *Department of Hematology, Pommeranian Academy of Medicine, Szcecin, Poland*

ANTHONY J. RAFFO, PhD • *Department of Medicine, College of Physicians and Surgeons, Columbia University, New York, NY*

JEAN-SERGE REMY, PhD • *Laboratoire de Chimie Génétique Associé CNRS, Faculte de Pharmacie, Université Louis Pasteur de Strasbourg, Illkirch, France*

JEAN PHILIPPE RICHARD, MSC • *UMR5124 CNRS, Institut de Genetique Moleculaire, Universite de Montpellier II, Montpellier, France*

FAYE A. ROGERS, PhD • *Departments of Therapeutic Radiology and Genetics, Yale University School of Medicine, New Haven, CT*

JOHN J. ROSSI, PhD • *Division of Molecular Biology, Beckman Research Institute of the City of Hope, Duarte, CA*

GEORG SCZAKIEL, PhD • *Institute for Molecular Medicine, University of Lübeck, Lübeck, Germany*

SUSAN E. SHETZLINE, PhD • *Department of Medicine, University of Pennsylvania School of Medicine, Philadelphia, PA*

C. A. STEIN, MD, PhD • *Department of Medical Oncology/Medicine, Albert Einstein College of Medicine, Bronx, NY*

LUN-QUAN SUN, PhD • *Johnson & Johnson Research Laboratories, Sydney, Australia*

ERIC VIVÈS, PhD • *UMR5124 CNRS, Institut de Genetique Moleculaire, Universite de Montpellier II, Montpellier, France*

JENS M. WARNECKE, PhD • *Institute for Molecular Medicine, University of Lübeck, Lübeck, Germany*

ZUO ZHANG, PhD • *Cold Spring Harbor Laboratory, Cold Spring Harbor, NY*

GUY ZUBER, PhD • *Laboratoire de Chimie Génétique Associé CNRS, Faculte de Pharmacie, Université Louis Pasteur de Strasbourg, Illkirch, France*

I | INTRODUCTION AND PERSPECTIVE

1

Antisense Methodology
An Assessment After 25 Years

Fritz Eckstein, PhD

CONTENTS

1. INTRODUCTION

The original concept for antisense methodology for the sequence-dependent inhibition of gene expression was remarkably simple. An oligonucleotide (ODN) complementary to a region of an mRNA to form a complex should prevent the ribosome from traveling along the message and thus prevent translation *(1)*. Now, with 25 years of experience, we realize that we have overlooked a fair number of problems associated with this strategy. However, this time has not been wasted, as it has given us insight into questions that were not anticipated. Therefore the development of the strategy was, and probably still is, an interesting and challenging learning process. The literature of the antisense field is immense, and many reviews have dealt with the potential for application and the difficulties encountered *(2–6)*. This chapter briefly discusses the areas where progress has been made over the years.

From: *Cancer Drug Discovery and Development:*
Nucleic Acid Therapeutics in Cancer
Edited by: A. M. Gewirtz © Humana Press Inc., Totowa, NJ

2. BASIC REQUIREMENTS FOR THE TECHNOLOGY

Various requirements have to be fulfilled for an ODN to be effective in the inhibition of gene expression. Such an ODN must have high stability against degradation by nucleases and obviously has to be able to bind to the mRNA to form a stable complex. ODN-accessible sites on the target RNA have to be identified for annealing. Subsequently, this complex has to be susceptible to degradation of the RNA part by RNase H, although certain ODN analogues operate in an RNase H-independent manner. Finally, the ODN of choice must be transportable into cells efficiently. In all these areas considerable progress has been made over the years, contributing to the success of the antisense methodology.

3. MECHANISM

The mechanism of inhibition of gene expression by the most commonly used phosphorothioate ODNs is most likely due to the degradation of the target mRNA by RNase H in the RNA–ODN complex. This assumption rests mainly on the observation that ODNs with modifications that interfere with the action of RNase H do not show the anticipated inhibition of expression. There is as yet no direct proof that RNase H is essential, but the data are consistent with that notion.

Activation of RNase H demands a DNA-like or B-conformation of the ODN. This requirement is obviously best met by oligodeoxynucleotides because they are present in this conformation. However, DNA–RNA complexes are not as stable as RNA–RNA complexes, which makes ODN with an RNA-like or A-conformation more desirable for hybridization with RNA. Thus, there is a dilemma in that one conformation is most suitable for one of the desired properties, which is, unfortunately, not optimal for the other *(7)*.

There is an interesting concern with the ODN phosphorothioate analogues a separate class of molecules *(8,9)*. These ODNs are generally synthesized as a pair of diastereomers and the question arises whether both diastereomers have the same ability to support the RNase H reaction (Fig. 1). The Stec laboratory had designed a stereospecific synthesis for the two diastereomers and could therefore test this question *(10)*. It was found that the Rp diastereomer infers the higher thermal stability on complex formation and also results in higher RNase H activity. Yet, the Sp diastereomer was more stable against nuclease degradation and resulted in better inhibition of gene expression followed closely by the mixture of diastereomers. Thus, at least for the phosphorothioates stability apparently is the more decisive factor for the efficiency of inhibition of expression. This is a nice example of the compromises one has to settle for when trying to optimize even a simple part of the whole antisense machinery.

With RNase H presumably as an integral part of the mechanism, the ODNs do not act stoechiometrically but after product dissociation can induce another round of RNase H cleavage. Thus it can be looked at as a catalytic process that lowers

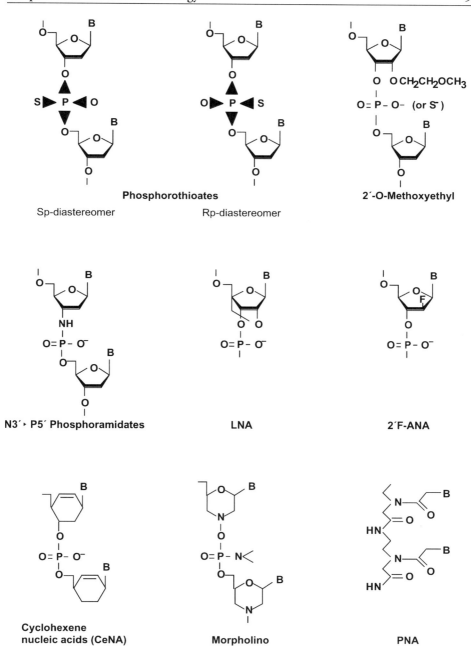

Fig. 1. Structures of oligonucleotides used in antisense methodology.

the required concentration of ODN. Once the mRNA is cleaved, the two products are believed to be degraded by subsequent action of nucleases. There is, however, an interesting observation in several cell lines that the 3' product can be stable and even be translated to proteins devoid of the N-terminus *(11)*. Whether this is a special case for a particular sequence context, for example, or more general will have to be seen.

One complication with respect to the sequence specificity of the antisense effect can be that RNase H is satisfied for cleavage with a short stretch of nucleotide complementarity. This can result in cleavage of RNAs of closely related members of a protein family with identical sequences in the region that has been chosen for the ODN docking. This has been exemplified for the protein kinase C family *(4)*.

4. STABILITY

One of the first problems to be identified as an obstacle for efficient performance of ODNs in inhibiting gene expression was the short lifetime of ordinary ODNs because of degradation by nucleases. This was solved for the first generation of ODNs by the introduction of phosphorothioate linkages *(8,9,12–14)*). The reason why the phosphorothioates are less susceptible to nucleases is only now becoming apparent. As aforementioned, the chemical synthesis of the phosphorothioate ODNs results in a mixture of diastereomers, unless methods for stereospecific syntheses are applied. Brautigam et al. demonstrated the consequences of enzyme–phosphorothioate interaction in an elegant X-ray structural analysis of the 3'–5' exonuclease of the Klenow polymerase in a complex with an oligonucleotide *(15)*. Of the two phosphorothioate diastereomers of the last internucleotidic linkage at the 3' end, only the Rp diastereomer is cleaved, whereas the Sp is resistant to cleavage. In the structure with the Rp diastereomer, the two essential metal ions at the active site of the enzyme are positioned very similarly as with the phosphate substrate. However, for the Sp phosphorothioate, both these metal ions are displaced by the larger van der Waals radius of sulfur as compared to oxygen, explaining the resistance to cleavage of this diastereomer. Similar arguments for resistance of phosphorothioate substrates can presumably be made for other nucleases even if they do not contain metal ions at the active site, simply by displacing essential functional groups by the somewhat larger sulfur than oxygen. This larger size would interfere with the proper positioning of functional groups in an 180-degree alignment of the nucleophile and the leaving group essential for cleavage *(8)*. Because the active site of an enzyme is chiral, the interaction for the two diastereomers will differ, and thus a mixture of diastereomers as normally employed is an advantage.

The initial enthusiasm for phosphorothioates was dampened by the realization later that this modification renders the oligodeoxynucleotides "sticky" for proteins, particularly those that normally associate with highly negatively charged molecules such as heparin *(4,16)*. A certain sequence and length dependence can be observed in these interactions, which might not only be responsible for cytotoxicity but could also interfere with gene expression in an antisense-independent manner. Interestingly, the question why phosphorothioate oligonucleotides should be more affine to proteins than their phosphate parents has not been solved as yet *(8,14)*.

5. GAPMERS

A logical consequence of the complications encountered with the phosphorothioate modification as mentioned above was to reduce the number of phosphorothioates in an ODN without compromising nuclease resistance. This was first addressed by designing ODNs where only the central part of 5–10 nucleotides contains phosphorothioates but the flanks consist of 2'-modified nucleotides, the so-called gapmers or mixed backbone ODNs. These modifications are incompatible with RNase H activity but the central part would still support enzymatic cleavage of target RNA after annealing. A stretch of a few nucleotides is all that is required by the enzyme to cleave the RNA *(17)*. Protection of the flanks is most often achieved by introduction of 2'-*O*-methyl or 2'-methoxyethyl groups, which also render the flanks less susceptible to nucleases (Fig. 1) *(18,19)*. Additionally, the 2'-*O*-modification lets the ODN adopt the RNA-like conformation, resulting in better hybridization thermodynamics of the ODN than if consisting purely of deoxynucleotides. However, although the nuclease stability inferred by these modifications seems sufficient for cell culture experiments, in vivo applications still require phosphorothioates even in the flanks. Interestingly, the phosphorothioates in conjunction with the 2'-modification apparently do not elicit the undesired interactions with proteins. The reason for this is unclear at present. An example for the potential of such phosphorothioate gapmers is the inhibition of Fas expression in mice for the protection against fulminant hepatitis *(19)*. Clinical trials with gapmers have not been reported so far.

Structural elements that are compatible with RNase H are still not well understood. For example, modified oligonucleotides such as locked nucleic acids (LNA) *(20)*, *cyc*lohexene nucleic acids (CeNA) *(21)*, and 2'-fluoroarabinonucleotides (2'-F-ANA) *(22)* do sustain this enzymatic activity to various degrees (Fig. 1). These analogs, like the 2'-*O*-alkylated oligoribonucleotides, adopt an RNA-like (A-form) conformation, assuring high binding affinities for the RNA target. Additionally, they are resistant to nucleases. Thus, they combine a number of favorable attributes to be excellently suited for the antisense strategy. So far, these analogues have not been extensively tested yet for the inhibition of gene expression in cell culture or in vivo. It is therefore too premature to estimate their full potential and to predict whether they represent alternatives to the phosphoro-thioate ODNs.

There are, however, antisense-ODNs that do not induce RNase H activity but nevertheless can interfere with gene expression. These are, for example, N3'–P5'-phosphoramidate oligonucleotides *(23)*, peptide nucleic acids (PNA) *(24)*, and morpholino oligonucleotides *(25)* (Fig. 1). The latter two, because of lack of negative charges on the backbone, cannot be taken up by cells with cationic carriers as it is normally done, at least for cell culture experiments. They require cell scraping or, as shown for PNA, conjugation with cationic peptides to facili-tate cellular uptake *(26)*. The inhibitory activity of these RNase H-inactive ODNs is presumably based on the action as physical blocks for the movement of the ribosome to result in translational arrest. However, one might keep an open mind for alternative mechanisms.

At present the most frequently used and the furthest developed, ODNs are the phosphorothioate-containing ODNs, either as purely deoxynucleotides or as gapmers. There are extensive data that indicate they can interfere with gene expression in cell culture as well as in vivo, and clinical trials are in progress. Examples are antisense-ODNs directed against Bcl-2 *(16,27,28)* or against pro-tein kinase C-α *(29)*.

6. IMMUNOSTIMULATION

An interesting complication arises from the effect of CpG dinucleotides within an ODN. Several types of immune cells possess pattern recognition receptors that can distinguish prokaryotic from vertebrate DNA on the basis of unmethylated CpG dinucleotides in the former. Bacterial or synthetic ODNs containing these CpG motifs can activate such responses, which include activation of B cells, den-dritic cells, macrophages, and natural killer cells *(30)*. Such ODN induce innate immunity and have great promise as adjuvants for vaccination and as immuno-therapeutics for allergic diseases and cancer. The optimal motif for driving human B-cell activation is the sequence GTCGTT. These ODNs are also applied as phosphorothioates, but because they act at very low concentrations, the often encountered undesired side effects of the phosphorothioates are not observed.

Many antisense ODNs contain such a CpG motif and thus might exert their effect by the immunostimulation rather than by a antisense effect alone. The two effects are usually difficult to disentangle. However, testing for the absence of typical effects associated with immune stimulation can strengthen the argument for a purely antisense effect *(28)*. As long as the CpG dinucleotide is part of the 2'-modified flanks of the ODN, immunostimulation might not be involved, but this remains to be investigated. The work by Zhang et al. for the inhibition of Fas expression in mice where the CpG is contained in the modified flank would support this reasoning *(19)*. In this instance, a single mutation distant from the

CpG in the ODN abolished the antisense effect, indeed suggesting that immunostimulation is not triggered by the modified CpG.

7. SITE SELECTION

Part of the failure initially to achieve positive results with antisense ODNs was that not much thought had been given to the accessibility of ODNs to the target RNA, not worrying about mRNA secondary structure. However, it transpired through walking of ODNs along an mRNA that there are noticeable differences in the degree of inhibition depending on the site of ODN-annealing *(31,32)*. This observation stimulated the search for experimental and computational approaches for the identification of such optimal sites. The most commonly used experimental analysis is annealing of a totally randomized ODN of about 10 nucleotides in length to the transcript in question and incubation with RNase H *(33,34)*. The question of course arises whether RNA sites identified by scanning of the transcript are also accessible on the mRNA in the intracellular environment. Thus, Scherr et al. have extended this method to analyze RNA in cellular extracts that should be more similar to the in vivo situation *(35)*. They show that a computer-aided approach is consistent with experimental studies in cell extracts. An interesting analysis for accessible sites has been pursued by the Southern laboratory with oligonucleotide arrays *(36)*. Interpretation of these data have been used in an attempt to understand the mechanism of ODN binding to transcripts. Some principles do emerge such that all sites contain a single-stranded region and an adjacent stem to accommodate the ODN to form a coaxial stack. However, we are still far away from fully understanding the structural and thermodynamic requirements for optimal annealing. The chemical nature of the ODN might also play a role in this process *(37)*. The question of how far annealing and cleavage data obtained by any of these methods translate reliably into the in vivo situation has to await further investigations.

8. ALTERNATIVE STRATEGIES

Although the ODN strategy of sequence-specific inhibition of gene expression was the first to be conceived, it has not remained the only one. Ribozymes also permit specific cleavage of RNA *(38–40)*. The appealing feature of the ribozyme-based strategy is the ribozyme's inherent catalytic activity, which does not require the action of an enzyme for RNA cleavage. Another difference with the ODN method is the ribozyme-based strategy's alternative way of application, as the ribozyme sequence can be incorporated in a vector for intracellular transient or even stable transcription. Several publications document the success of the ribozyme approach by either method of application, and clinical trials are under way. Against all expectations, also, DNAzymes could be selected *(41)*. This was surprising, because most had attributed the catalytic activity to RNA to its higher flexibility and to an advantage through the additional 2'-OH group. Therefore, the catalytic activity of DNA came as a surprise even more so as the most active showed better cleavage activities than ribozymes, which was also demonstrated in a direct comparison (42). Interestingly, chemical functionality can be incorporated into the DNAzymes by the use of base-modified nucleotides in the selection process to enhance cleavage activity (43). DNAzymes have been studied in various systems for inhibition of gene expression (44,45). Not surprisingly, they require modification for increased stability against nuclease degradation, and phosphorothioates can be one of the choices (46). However, considerably more testing, particularly in animal models, has to be done to evaluate the full potential of DNAzymes.

More recently, RNA interference has joined the armamentarium for sequence specific inhibition of gene expression (47). Short, double-stranded, synthetic oligoribonucleotides, or those produced by intracellular processing of double-stranded RNA, induce cleavage of the target mRNA at very low concentrations, as shown not only in cell culture but also in cell extracts and in lower animals such as *Drosophila* and *C. elegans*. It is assumed that some mechanism of amplification of the oligoribonucleotides is responsible for the requirement of such low concentrations (48). Interestingly, the accessibility of oligoribonucleotides to the mRNA is much less restricted, so an elaborate search for suitable target sites is not necessary. RNA interference has been successfully extented to murine cell types of embryonic origin where the double stranded RNA was stably expressed. The method remains to be tested in adult animals (49).

9. CONCLUSION

There is no doubt that the antisense strategy has encountered many unanticipated problems. This, however, might not be surprising because this approach represents the development of an entirely new class of compounds to be introduced into cells. Given that the cell contains a finely tuned machinery of proteins, nucleic acids, lipids, and carbohydrates where the components are compartmentalized, directing negatively charged oligonucleotides to the desired target, without interfering with any other component, is like running an obstacle course. The success of the antisense strategy as it stands today is a marvelous example for collaboration among chemists, biochemists, and cell biologists. These interdisciplinary efforts continue and might generate oligonucleotides of different structures with superior qualities for the antisense method. Meanwhile, it is hoped that the ongoing clinical trials with existing ODNs will result in the appearance of therapeutic drugs to culminate a long and burdensome journey (50).

REFERENCES

1. Zamecnik PC, Stephenson ML. Inhibition of Rous sarcoma virus replication and transformation by a specific oligonucleotide. Proc Natl Acad Sci USA 1978; 75:285–288.
2. Cook ST. (ed.) Antisense drug technology: Principles, strategies, and application. Marcel Dekker, New York, 2001.
3. Tamm I, Dörken B, Hartmann G. Antisense therapy in oncology: new hope for an old idea? Lancet 2002; 358:489–497.
4. Lebedeva I, Stein CA. Antisense oligonucleotides: promise and reality. Annu Rev Pharmacol Toxicol 2001; 41:403–419.
5. Agrawal S, Kandimalla ER. Antisense and/or immunostimulatory oligonucleotide therapeutics. Curr Cancer Drug Targets 2001; 1:197–209.
6. Gewirtz A. Suppression of gene expression by targeted disruption of messenger RNA: Available options and current strategies. Stem Cells 2000; 18:307–319.
7. Kvaerno L, Wengel J. Antisense molecules and furanose conformations—is it really that simple? Chem Commun 2001;1419–1424.
8. Eckstein F. Nucleoside phosphorothioates. Annu Rev Biochem 1985; 54:367–402.
9. Verma S, Eckstein F. Modified oligonucleotides: Synthesis and strategy for users. Annu Rev Biochem 1998; 67:99–134.
10. Stec WJ, Cierniewski CS, Okruszek A, et al. Stereodependent inhibition of plasminogen activator inhibitor type 1 by phosphorothioate oligonucleotides: Proof of sequence specificity in cell culture and in vivo rat experiments. Antisense & Nucleic Acid Drug Dev 1997; 7:57–573.
11. Thoma C, Hasselblatt P, Köck J, et al. Generation of stable mRNA fragments and translation of N-truncated proteins induced by antisense oligodeoxynucleotides. Mol Cell 2001; 8:865–872.
12. Matsukura M, Shinozuka K, Zon G, et al. Phosphorothioate analogues of oligodeoxy-nucleotides: Inhibitors of replication and cytopathic effects of human immunodeficiency virus. Proc Natl Acad Sci USA 1987; 84:7706–7710.
13. Agrawal S, Goodchild J, Civeira MP, Thornton AH, Sarin PS, Zamecnik PC. Oligodeoxynucleoside phosphoramidates and phosphorothioates as inhibitors of human immunodeficiency virus. Proc Natl Acad Sci USA 1988; 85:7079–7083.
14. Eckstein F. Phosphorothioate oligodeoxynucleotides: what is their origin and what is unique about them? Antisense & Nucleic Acid Drug Devel 2000; 10:117–121.
15. Brautigam CA, Steitz TA. Structural principles for the inhibition of the 3'–5' exonuclease activity of Escherichia coli DNA polymerase I by phosphorothioates. J Mol Biol 1998; 277:363–377.
16. Waters JS, Webb A, Cunningham D, et al. Phase I clinical and pharmacokinetic study of bcl-2 antisense oligonucleotide therapy in patients with non-Hodgkin's lymphoma. J Clin Oncol 2000; 18: 1812–1823.
17. Monia BP, Lesnik EA, Gonzalez C, et al. Evaluation of 2'-modified oligonucleotides containing 2'-deoxy gaps as antisense inhibitors of gene expression. J Biol Chem 1993; 268:14514–14522.
18. Ruskowski M, Qu T, Roskey A, Agrawal S. Biodistribution and metabolism of a mixed backbone oligonucleotide (GEM 231) following single and multiple dose administration in mice. Antisense & Nucleic Acid Drug Dev 2000; 10:333–345.
19. Zhang H, Cook J, Nickel J, et al. Reduction of liver Fas expression by an antisense oligonucleotide protects mice from fulminant hepatitis. Nature Biotechnol 2000; 18:862–867.
20. Wahlestedt C, Salmi P, Good L, et al. Potent and nontoxic antisense oligonucleotides containing locked nucleic acids. Proc Natl Acad Sci USA 2000; 97:5633–5638.
21. Verbeure B, Lescrinier E, Wang J, Herdewijn P. RNase H mediated cleavage of RNA by cyclohexene nucleic acid (CeNA). Nucleic Acids Res 2001; 29:4941–4947.

22. Wilds CJ, Damha MJ. 2'-Deoxy-2'-fluoro-β-D-arabinonucleosides and oligonucleotides (2'F-ANA): synthesis and physicochemical studies. Nucleic Acids Res 2000; 28:3625–3635.
23. Gryaznov SM. Oligonucleotide N3'–P5' phosphoramidates as potential therapeutic agents. Biochim Biophys Acta 1999; 1489:131–140.
24. Nielsen PE. Peptide nucleic acids as therapeutic agents. Curr Opin Struct Biol 1999; 9:353–357.
25. Hudziak RM, Summerton J, Weller DD, Iversen PL. Antiproliferative effects of steric blocking phosphordiamidate morpholino antisense agents directed against c-myc. Antisense & Nucleic Acid Drug Dev 2000; 10:163–176.
26. Eriksson M, Nielsen PE, Good L. Cell permeabilization and uptake of antisense peptide-nucleic acid (PNA) into Escherichia coli. J Biol Chem 2002; 277:7144–7147.
27. Zangemeister-Wittke U, Leech SH, Olie RA, et al. A novel *bis*pecific antisense oligonucleotide inhibiting both bcl-2 and bcl-xL expression efficiently induces apoptosis in tumor cells. Clin Cancer Res 2000; 6:2547–2555.
28. Jansen B, Wacheck V, Heere-Ress E, et al. Chemosensitisation of malignant melanoma by BCL2 antisense therapy. Lancet 2000; 356:1728–1733.
29. Yuen AR, Halsey J, Fisher GA, et al. Phase I clinical study of an antisense oligonucleotide to protein kinase C-α (ISIS 3521/CGP 64128A) in patients with cancer. Clin Cancer Res 1999; 5:3357–3363.
30. Krieg A. From bugs to drugs: therapeutic immunomodulation with oligodeoxynucleotides containing CpG sequences from bacterial DNA. Antisense & Nucleic Acid Drug Devel 2001; 11:181–188.
31. Peyman A, Helsberg M, Kretzschmar G, Mag M, Grabley S, Uhlmann E. Inhibition of viral growth by antisense oligonucleotides directed against the IE110 and the UL mRNA of Herpes Simplex virus type-1. Biol Chem Hoppe-Seyler 1995; 376:195–198.
32. Monia BP, Johnston JF, Geiger T, Muller M, Fabbro D. Antitumor activity of a phosphorothioate antisense oligodeoxynucleotide targeted against C-raf kinase. Nat Medicine 1996; 2:669–675.
33. Ho SP, Bao Y, Lesher T, et al. Mapping of RNA accessible sites for antisense experiment with oligonucleotide libraries. Nat. Biotechnol. 1998: 16:59–63.
34. Birikh KR, Berlin YA, Soreq H, Eckstein F. Probing accessible sites for ribozymes on human acetylcholinesterase RNA. RNA 1997; 3:429–437.
35. Scherr M, Rossi JJ, Sczakiel G, Patzel V. RNA accessibility prediction: a theoretical approach is consistent with experimental studies in cell extracts. Nucleic Acids Res 2000; 28:2455–2461.
36. Sohail M, Hochegger H, Klotzbücher A, et al. Antisense oligonucleotides selected by hybridization to scanning arrays are effective reagents in vivo. Nucleic Acids Res 2001; 29:2041–2051.
37. Vickers TA, Wyatt JR, Freier SM. Effects of RNA secondary structure on cellular antisense activity. Nucleic Acids Res 2000; 28:1340–1347.
38. Bramlage B, Eckstein F. The hammerhead ribozyme. Biopolymers (Nucleic Acid Sciences) 2001; 52:147–154.
39. Pavco PA, Bouhana KS, Gallegos AM, et al. Antitumor and antimetastatic activity of ribozymes targeting the messenger RNA of vascular endothelial growth factor receptors. Clinical Cancer Res 2000; 6:2094–2103.
40. Rossi JJ. Therapeutic ribozymes. BioDrugs 1998; 1:1–10.
41. Santoro SW, Joyce GF. A general-purpose RNA-cleaving DNA enzyme. Proc Natl Acad Sci USA 1997; 94:4262–4266.
42. Kurreck J, Bieber B, Jahnel R, Erdmann VA. Comparative study of DNA enzymes and ribozymes against the same full length messenger RNA of the vanilloid receptor. J Biol Chem 2002; 277:7099–7107.
43. Santoro SW, Joyce GF, Sakthivel K, Gramatikova S, Barbas CF. RNA cleavage by a DNA enzyme with extended chemical functionality. J Am Chem Soc 2000; 122:2433–2439.

44. Santiago FS, Lowe HC, Kavurma MM, et al. New DNA enzyme targeting Egr-1 mRNA inhibits vascular smooth muscle proliferation and regrowth after injury. Nat Medicine 1999; 11:1264–1269.
45. Warashina M, Kuwabara T, Nakamatsu Y, Taira K. Extremely high and specific activity of DNA enzymes in cells with a Philadelphia chromosome. Chem Biol 1999; 6:237–250.
46. Sioud M, Leirdal M. Design of nuclease resistant protein kinase Cα DNA enzymes with potential therapeutic application. J Mol Biol 2000; 296:937–947.
47. Elbashir SM, Harborth J, Lendecke W, Yalcin A, Weber K, Tuschl T. Duplexes of 21-nucleotide RNAs mediate RNA interference in cultured mammalian cells. Nature 2001; 411:494–498.
48. Lipardi C., Wie Q, Paterson BM. RNAi as random degradative PCR: siRNA primers concert mRNA into dsRNA that are degraded to generate new siRNAs. Cell 2001; 107:297–307.
49. Paddison PJ, Caudy AA, Hannon GJ. Stable suppression of gene expression by RNAi in mammalian cells. Proc Natl Acad Sci USA 2002; 99:1443–1448.
50. Dove A. Antisense and sensibility. Nat Biotechnol 2002; 20:21–124.

2 Nucleic Acid Therapeutics
An Introduction

Alan M. Gewirtz, MD

CONTENTS

1. INTRODUCTION

The development of simple, reliable tools for modifying gene expression "on demand" would represent a major technical advance for cell biologists. Because much progress has been made in understanding the molecular pathogenesis of many diseases, we may easily hypothesize that these same tools could be of tremendous importance to clinicians as well. For example, many genes responsible for cellular transformation have been identified. If the function of these genes were shown to be either completely or relatively tumor specific, they would become legitimate targets for therapeutic manipulation of their expression. More effective, less toxic cancer treatments could reasonably be expected to result if the strategy were successful.

The notion that gene expression could be modified through use of exogenous nucleic acids derives from studies by Paterson et al., who first used single-stranded DNA to inhibit translation of a complementary RNA in a cell free system in 1977 (1). The following year, Zamecnik and Stephenson showed that a short (13mer) DNA oligodeoxynucleotide antisense to the Rous sarcoma virus could inhibit viral replication in culture (2). Based on this work, the latter investigators are widely credited for having first suggested the therapeutic utility of antisense nucleic acids. In the mid-1980s, the existence of naturally occurring antisense RNAs and their role in regulating gene expression was demonstrated (3–5). These observations were particularly important because they lent credibility to the belief that "antisense" was more than a laboratory phenomenon and

From: *Cancer Drug Discovery and Development:*
Nucleic Acid Therapeutics in Cancer
Edited by: A. M. Gewirtz © Humana Press Inc., Totowa, NJ

encouraged belief in the hypothesis that reverse complementary ASNA could be utilized in living cells to manipulate gene expression. These seminal papers, and the many that have since followed, have stimulated the development of technologies employing nucleic acids to manipulate gene expression. As discussed immediately below, virtually all available methods rely on some type of nucleotide sequence recognition for targeting specificity but differ where and how they perturb the flow of genetic information.

Strategies for modulating gene expression may be thought of as being either "anti-gene" or anti-mRNA, reviewed in (6,7). Anti-gene strategies focus primarily on gene targeting by homologous recombination (8,9), or by triple-helix-forming oligodeoxynucleotides (TFOs) (10,11). Because homologous recombination involves vector technology and, at least at the present time, is much too inefficient for clinical use, it is not considered further in this discussion. TFOs bind in the major groove of duplex DNA in a sequence-specific manner (11). Gene targeting with these molecules is constrained by the fact that TFOs require runs of purines on one strand and pyrimidines on the other (~10–30 nts in length) for stable hybridization. The TFO can be composed of either polypurine or polypyrimidine bases, but hybridization always occurs on the purine strand of the duplex through formation of Hoogsteen bonds (Fig. 1).

Although successful use of this strategy for blocking transcription and inducing specific mutations in vitro and in vivo has been reported, the frequency of such events is considerably less than 1%, and therefore this approach is also too inefficient for clinical use at this time.

ASNA transcription factor decoy molecules have also been employed to disrupt gene expression at the level of transcription (12). For many technical reasons, including limited gene accessibility within the nuclear/chromosomal structure, the clinical application of these methods has not progressed at a very rapid rate. An alternative approach, using polyamides, or lexitropsins, has been described by Kielkopf and colleagues (13–15). Polyamide ligands contain the aromatic amino acids pyrrole (Py), hydroxypyrrole (Hp), and imidazole (Im). These small molecules have the ability to diffuse into the nucleus where they can then contact double-stranded DNA in the minor groove. Pairs of such amino acids can be constructed that recognize all four Watson-Crick basepairs. It is theoretically possible then to construct polyamides that will recognize specific DNA sequences and squelch gene expression by preventing transcription in a manner analogous to TFOs (see Fig. 2).

However, these small molecules also share problems in common with TFOs. Included among these is the fact that recognition of longer sequences, as would be required for gene-specific recognition, require larger molecules, which are likely to have trouble gaining access to the nucleosome. In addition, maintaining the appropriate amino acid register for accurate sequence recognition is also a significant issue (17). Accordingly, much remains to be accomplished by the

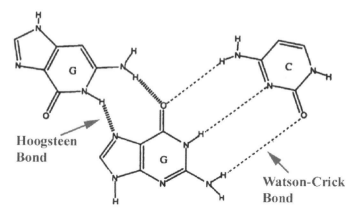

Fig.1. Triple helix formation at nucleotide level showing Watson-Crick and Hoogsteen Bond formation between duplex pairs and the third strand.

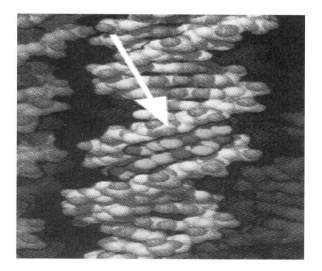

Fig. 2. Lexitropsin (polymide) molecule (arrow) binding in minor groove of DNA (adapted from ref. *16*).

scientists interested in this approach before attempts at clinical use can be contemplated.

A larger body of work has focused on destabilizing mRNA. This approach, although less favorable than antigene strategies from a stoichiometric point of view, is nonetheless attractive because mRNA, unlike a given gene's DNA, is theoretically accessible to attack while being transcribed, transported from the nucleus, and translated. Two ASNA-based strategies have emerged for blocking translation. One employs oligonucleotides that act as alternate binding sites, or "decoys," for proteins that act as transcriptional activators, or as stabilizing elements that normally interact with a given mRNA *(18,19)*. By attracting away the desired protein, the decoy may prevent transcription or induce instability, and ultimately destruction, of the mRNA. The use of decoy RNAs for therapeutic purposes was initially suggested by Baltimore in 1988 *(20)*. The approach has gained credibility since the molecules are nontoxic and appear to have been successful for control of viral gene expression, including HIV, in vitro *(21,22)*. It is assumed in these studies that the decoy is directly interfering with HIV replication by sequestering REV, but this was not formally proven *(21)*. Its mechanism of action is therefore uncertain. Recent studies on human β-globin mRNA are of interest in this regard. Stability determinants for this mRNA species have been defined in sufficient detail so that it can be used as a model system for testing the hypothesis that altering mRNA stability with decoys will be a useful form of therapy *(23–25)*.

The other strategy for destabilizing mRNA is the more widely applied antisense strategy, using ribozymes, DNAzymes, antisense RNA, or antisense DNA (ODN). This approach to gene squelching has been the subject of numerous authoritative reviews *(6,26,27)*, but simply stated, delivering an antisense nucleic acid into a cell where the gene of interest is expressed should lead to hybridization between the antisense sequence and the targeted gene's mRNA. Stable mRNA-antisense duplexes cannot be translated, and depending on the chemical composition of the antisense molecule, can lead to the destruction of the mRNA by binding of endogenous nucleases, such as RNase H, or by intrinsic enzymatic activity engineered into the sequence (ribozymes and DNAzymes) (*see* Fig. 3).

Finally, a third and newly developing approach for targeting mRNA is called post-transcriptional gene silencing, or RNA interference (RNAi) *(28,29)* (Fig. 4). RNAi is the process by which double-stranded RNA (dsRNA) targets mRNA for destruction in a sequence-dependent manner. The mechanism of RNAi involves processing of dsRNA into 21–23 basepair (bp) fragments that hybridize with the target mRNA and initiate its destruction. The mechanism for RNAi is fast being elucidated, although many intriguing questions remain to be answered *(28)*. At this time, it appears likely that dsRNA is processed by an enzyme called Dicer *(30–32)* into approx 21–22 nt long double strands. These small cleavage products are then incorporated into a larger RnP complex that simultaneously scans the complementary mRNA sequence for homology to the small, now un- wound, RNA fragment and then promotes its destruction through an enzymes integral to the complex *(33–35)*. RNAi has been employed successfully for gene silencing in a variety of experimental systems including petunias, tobacco plants, neurospora, *C. elegans*, insects, planaria, hydra, zebrafish. The use of long

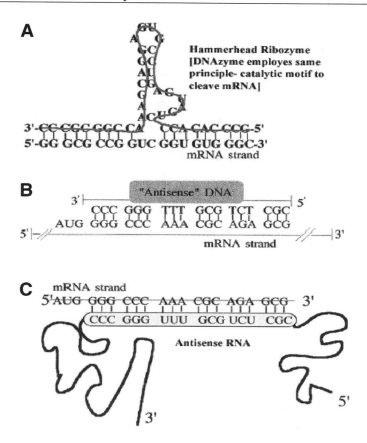

Fig. 3. Antisense strategies for squelching gene expression.

dsRNA to squelch expression in mammalian cells has been tried, largely without success *(36)*. It has been suggested that mammalian cells recognize these sequences as invading pathogens, which triggers an interferon response that leads to apoptosis and cell death *(37)*. However, a number of recent reports suggest that RNA double strands of approx 21–22 nts in length, called short interfering RNA (siRNA), may be able to squelch expression in mammalian somatic cells if appropriately modified to contain 3'-hydroxy and 5'-phosphate groups *(38–41)*. Although reports about the utility of this method for silencing mammalian genes continue to accumulate *(42–45)*, the ability to apply this method to all types of mammalian cells remains uncertain *(36)*. This is also true for traditional antisense experiments, and not surprisingly, the possibility of experimental artifacts being misinterpreted as specific gene targeting is being increasingly recognized as well *(46)*. Accordingly, it is highly likely that many

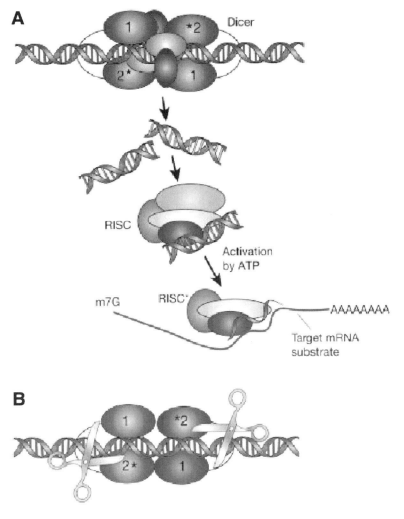

Fig. 4. Hypothetical RNAi mechanism (adapted from ref. *41*).

technical issues related to employing nucleic acid therapeutics in general will also apply to siRNA, including the need to identify mRNA accessible sequences in a predictable way *(47)*.

The power of nucleic-acid-mediated gene squelching has been demonstrated in experiments in which critical biological information has been gathered, and subsequently confirmed, using alternative or complementary experimental methods including the critical role of the *c-myb* gene in hematopoietic cell proliferation. These experiments were the motivation for an early example of "bench-to-bedside" research as they culminated in some of the first phase I/II antisense oligodeoxynucleotide studies for the treatment of leukemia here at the University of Pennsylvania *(48)*. A major conclusion of the work is that, at the least, expression of the targeted gene (*c-myb*) could be abrogated under clinically relevant conditions.

Nevertheless, despite many successes *(48–50)*, it is widely appreciated that the ability of antisense nucleic acids to modify gene expression is variable, and therefore wanting, in terms of reliability *(51–53)*. Several issues have been implicated as root cause of this problem, including molecule delivery to targeted cells *(51)* and identification of hybridization accessible sequence *(6)*. Sequence accessibility is determined by mRNA folding, which in turn is dictated by internal basepairing and the proteins that associate with the RNA in a living cell. Attempts to accurately predict the in vivo structure of RNA have been fraught with difficulty *(54)*. Accordingly, mRNA targeting with any hybridization-dependent targeting vehicle, including siRNA *(47)*, is largely a random process, accounting for many experiments where the addition of an antisense nucleic acid yields no effect on expression.

Recent work from this laboratory suggests that the self-quenching reporter molecules (SQRM) that we are developing will be useful for solving in vivo RNA structure *(55)*.

Another significant problem in this field is the limited ability to deliver ASNA into cells and have them reach their target *(51)*. Without this ability, it is clear that even an appropriately targeted sequence is not likely to be efficient. As a general rule, oligonucleotides are taken up primarily through a combination of adsorptive and fluid-phase endocytosis *(56–59)*. After internalization, confocal and electron microscopy studies have indicated that the bulk of the oligonucleotides enter the endosome/lysosome compartment, where most of the material either becomes trapped or degraded. Biologic inactivity is the predictable result of these events. Nevertheless, oligonucleotides can escape from the vesicles intact, enter the cytoplasm, and then diffuse into the nucleus, where they presumably acquire their mRNA or, in the case of decoys, protein target. In the last few years, delivery technologies have improved considerably, and it is likely that these and other newly evolving technologies can be used to delivery optimized nucleic acids to their cellular targets.

It is our hypothesis that development of effectively targeted, and efficiently delivered, nucleic acid molecules will lead to important advances in the diagnosis and treatment of human malignancies *(48)*. As was true for the field of monoclonal antibody therapies, where hype was followed by disappointment and then finally genuine triumph of the concept, we believe that breakthroughs in the area of nucleic-acid-mediated gene squelching will shortly be forthcoming and will more than justify the time and resources expended in developing the therapeutic use of these molecules.

REFERENCES

1. Paterson BM, Roberts BE, Kuff EL. Structural gene identification and mapping by DNA-mRNA hybrid-arrested cell-free translation. Proc Natl Acad Sci USA 1977; 74(10):4370–4374.
2. Stephenson ML, Zamecnik PC. Inhibition of Rous sarcoma viral RNA translation by a specific oligodeoxyribonucleotide. Proc Natl Acad Sci USA 1978; 75(1): 285–288.
3. Simons RW, Kleckner N. Translational control of IS10 transposition. Cell 1983; 34(2): 683–691.
4. Izant JG, Weintraub H. Inhibition of thymidine kinase gene expression by anti-sense RNA: a molecular approach to genetic analysis. Cell 1984; 36(4):1007–1015.
5. Mizuno T, Chou MY, Inouye M. A unique mechanism regulating gene expression: translational inhibition by a complementary RNA transcript (micRNA). Proc Natl Acad Sci USA 1984; 81(7): 1966–1970.
6. Gewirtz AM, Sokol DL, Ratajczak MZ. Nucleic acid therapeutics: state of the art and future prospects. Blood 1998; 92(3):712–736.
7. Opalinska JB, Gewirtz AM. Nucleic-acid therapeutics: basic principles and recent applications. Nat Rev Drug Discov 2002; 1(7):503–514.
8. Melton DW. Gene targeting in the mouse. Bioessays 1994; 16(9):633–638.
9. Stasiak A. Getting down to the core of homologous recombination [comment]. Science 1996; 272(5263):828–829.
10. Helene C. Control of oncogene expression by antisense nucleic acids. Eur J Cancer 1994; 30A(11):1721–1726.
11. Knauert MP, Glazer PM. Triplex forming oligonucleotides: sequence-specific tools for gene targeting. Hum Mol Genet 2001; 10(20):2243–2251.
12. Sharma HW, erez JR, Higgins-Sochaski K, Hsiao R, Narayanan R. Transcription factor decoy approach to decipher the role of NF-kappa B in oncogenesis. Anticancer Res 1996; 16(1):61–69.
13. Kielkopf CL, Baird EE, Dervan PB, Rees DC. Structural basis for G.C recognition in the DNA minor groove. Nat Struct Biol 1998; 5(2):104–109.
14. Kielkopf CL, White S, Szewczyk JW, et al. A structural basis for recognition of A.T and T.A base pairs in the minor groove of B-DNA. Science 1998; 282(5386):111–115.
15. Kielkopf CL, Bremer RE, White S, et al. Structural effects of DNA sequence on T.A recognition by hydroxypyrrole/pyrrole pairs in the minor groove. J Mol Biol 2000; 295(3):557–567.
16. Goodsell DS. The molecular perspective: DNA. Stem Cells 2000; 18(2):148–149.
17. Urbach AR, Dervan PB. Toward rules for 1:1 polyamide:DNA recognition. Proc Natl Acad Sci USA 2001; 98(8):4343–4348.
18. Beelman CA, Parker R. Degradation of mRNA in eukaryotes. Cell 1995; 81(2): 179–183.
19. Liebhaber SA. mRNA stability and the control of gene expression. Nucleic Acids Symp Ser 1997; 36:29–32.
20. Baltimore D. Gene therapy. Intracellular immunization [news]. Nature 1988; 335(6189):395–396.
21. Sullenger BA, Gallardo HF, Ungers GE, Gilboa E. Analysis of trans-acting response decoy RNA-mediated inhibition of human immunodeficiency virus type 1 transactivation. J Virol 1991; 65(12):6811–6816.
22. Bevec D, Volc-Platzer B, Zimmermann K, et al.. Constitutive expression of chimeric neo-Rev response element transcripts suppresses HIV-1 replication in human CD4+ T lymphocytes. Hum Gene Ther 1994; 5(2):193–201.
23. Weiss IM, Liebhaber, SA. Erythroid cell-specific mRNA stability elements in the alpha 2-globin 3' nontranslated region. Mol Cell Biol 1995; 15(5):2457–2465.
24. Wang X, Kiledjian M, Weiss IM, Liebhaber SA. Detection and characterization of a 3' untranslated region ribonucleoprotein complex associated with human alpha-globin mRNA stability [published erratum appears in Mol Cell Biol 1995 Apr;15(4):2331]. Mol Cell Biol 1995; 15(3):1769–1777.

25. Thisted T, Lyakhov DL, Liebhaber SA. Optimized RNA targets of two closely related triple KH domain proteins, heterogeneous nuclear ribonucleoprotein K and alphaCP-2KL, suggest distinct modes of RNA recognition. PG-17484-96. J Biol Chem 2001; 276(20):17484–17496.
26. Scanlon KJ, Ohta Y, Ishida H, et al. Oligonucleotide-mediated modulation of mammalian gene expression. Faseb J 1995; 9(13):1288–1296.
27. Stein CA. How to design an antisense oligodeoxynucleotide experiment: a consensus approach. Antisense Nucleic Acid Drug Dev 1998; 8(2):129–132.
28. Nishikura K. A short primer on RNAi: RNA-directed RNA polymerase acts as a key catalyst. Cell 2001; 107(4): 415–418.
29. Sharp PA. RNAi and double-strand RNA. Genes Dev 1999; 13(2):139–141.
30. Hutvagner G, McLachlan J, Pasquinelli AE, Balint E, Tuschl T, Zamore PD. A cellular function for the RNA-interference enzyme Dicer in the maturation of the let-7 small temporal RNA. Science 2001; 293(5531):834–838.
31. Ketting RF, et al. Dicer functions in RNA interference and in synthesis of small RNA involved in developmental timing in C. elegans. Genes Dev 2001; 15(20):2654–2659.
32. Nicholson RH, Nicholson AW. Molecular characterization of a mouse cDNA encoding Dicer, a ribonuclease III ortholog involved in RNA interference. Mamm Genome 2002; 13(2):67–73.
33. Hammond SM, Boetther S, Caudy AA, Kobaashi R, Hannon GJ. Argonaute2, a link between genetic and biochemical analyses of RNAi. Science 2001; 293(5532):1146–1150.
34. Williams RW, Rubin GM. ARGONAUTE1 is required for efficient RNA interference in Drosophila embryos. Proc Natl Acad Sci USA 2002; 99(10):6889–6894.
35. Martinez J, Patkaniowska A, Urlaub H, Luhrmann R, Tuschl T. Single-stranded antisense siRNAs guide target RNA cleavage in RNAi. Cell 2002; 110(5):563–574.
36. Yang S, Tutton S, Pierce E, Yoon K. Specific double-stranded RNA interference in undifferentiated mouse embryonic stem cells. Mol Cell Biol 2001; 21(22):7807–7816.
37. Bernstein E, Denli AM, Hannon GJ. The rest is silence. RNA, 2001; 7(11):1509–1521.
38. Yang D, Lu H, Erickson JW. Evidence that processed small dsRNAs may mediate sequence-specific mRNA degradation during RNAi in Drosophila embryos. Curr Biol 2000; 10(19):1191–200.
39. Zamore PD, Tuschl T, Sharp PA, Bartel DP. RNAi: double-stranded RNA directs the ATP-dependent cleavage of mRNA at 21 to 23 nucleotide intervals. Cell 2000; 101(1):25–33.
40. Elbashir SM, Martinez J, Patkaniowska A, Lndeckel W, Tuschl T. Functional anatomy of siRNAs for mediating efficient RNAi in Drosophila melanogaster embryo lysate. Embo J 2001; 20(23):6877–6888.
41. Hannon GJ. RNA interference. Nature 2002; 418(6894):244–251.
42. Yu JY, DeRuiter SL, Turner DL. RNA interference by expression of short-interfering RNAs and hairpin RNAs in mammalian cells. Proc Natl Acad Sci USA 2002; 99(9):6047–6052.
43. Donze O, Picard DL. RNA interference in mammalian cells using siRNAs synthesized with T7 RNA polymerase. Nucleic Acids Res 2002; 30(10):e46.
44. Sui G, Soohoo C, Affar el B, Gay F, et al. A DNA vector-based RNAi technology to suppress gene expression in mammalian cells. Proc Natl Acad Sci USA 2002; 99(8):5515–5520.
45. Paddison PJ, Caudy AA, bernstein E, Hannon GJ, Conklin DS. Short hairpin RNAs (shRNAs) induce sequence-specific silencing in mammalian cells. Genes Dev 2002; 16(8):948–958.
46. Lassus P, Rodriguez J, Lazebnik Y. Confirming Specificity of RNAi in mammalian cells. Sci STKE 2002; 147:PL13.
47. Holen T, Amarzguioui M, Wiiger MT, Babaie E, Prydz H. Positional effects of short interfering RNAs targeting the human coagulation trigger tissue factor. Nucleic Acids Res 2002; 30(8):1757–1766.

48. Luger SM, O'Brien SG, Ratajczak J, et al. Oligodeoxynucleotide-mediated inhibition of c-myb gene expression in autografted bone marrow: a pilot study. Blood 2002; 99(4):1150–1158.
49. Methia N, Louache F, Vainchenker W, Wendling F. Oligodeoxynucleotides antisense to the proto-oncogene c-mpl specifically inhibit in vitro megakaryocytopoiesis. Blood 1993; 82(5):1395–13401.
50. Webb A, Cunningham D, Cotter F, et al. BCL-2 antisense therapy in patients with non-Hodgkin lymphoma. Lancet 1997; 349(9059):1137–1141.
51. Gewirtz AM, Stein CA, Glazer PM. Facilitating oligonucleotide delivery: helping antisense deliver on its promise. Proc Natl Acad Sci USA 1996; 93(8):3161–3163.
52. Stein CA, Does antisense exist? Nat Med 1995; 1(11):1119–1121.
53. Wagner RW, Flanagan WM. Antisense technology and prospects for therapy of viral infections and cancer. Mol Med Today 1997; 3(1):31–38.
54. Baskerville S, Ellington AD. RNA structure. Describing the elephant. Curr Biol 1995; 5(2):120–123.
55. Sokol DL, Zhang X, Lu P. Gewirtz AM. Real time detection of DNA. RNA hybridization in living cells. Proc Natl Acad Sci USA, 1998; 95(20):11538–11543.
56. Yakubov LA, Deeva EA, Zarytova VF, et al. Mechanism of oligonucleotide uptake by cells: involvement of specific receptors? Proc Natl Acad Sci USA 1989; 86(17):6454–6458.
57. Beltinger C, et al. Binding, uptake, and intracellular trafficking of phosphorothioate-modified oligodeoxynucleotides. J Clin Invest 1995; 95(4):1814–1823.
58. Arima H, Aramaki Y, Tsuchiya S. Effects of oligodeoxynucleotides on the physicochemical characteristics and cellular uptake of liposomes. J Pharm Sci 1997; 86(4): 438–442.
59. Laktionov PP, Dazard JE, Vives E, et al. Characterisation of membrane oligonucleotide-binding proteins and oligonucleotide uptake in keratinocytes. Nucleic Acids Res 1999; 27(11):2315–2324.

II BASIC METHODOLOGY

3 Targeted Genome Modification Via Triple Helix Formation

Faye A. Rogers, PhD
and Peter M. Glazer, MD, PhD

CONTENTS

1. INTRODUCTION

Over the last few decades, tremendous strides have been made in the identification of defective genes known to cause or contribute to the initiation or progression of different diseases. This research has led to new and innovative therapies in the treatment of disease. Traditionally, most active drugs are inhibitors of proteins. However, in recent years synthetic oligonucleotides have been developed as a means to rationally design therapeutic agents that selectively modulate gene expression. The ability to modulate a chosen gene's function or expression for therapeutic use would be ideal to stimulate or restore the production of gene products whose absence leads to illness. For instance, the ability to correct or "repair" defective genes that are associated with inherited diseases would be of tremendous clinical value.

Modulation of gene expression using oligonucleotides has been targeted at different steps in the information transfer pathway from the gene to protein synthesis. Antisense oligonucleotides have been used to achieve gene regulation by targeting the translation of mRNA into the corresponding protein. In the antigene

From: *Cancer Drug Discovery and Development:*
Nucleic Acid Therapeutics in Cancer
Edited by: A. M. Gewirtz © Humana Press Inc., Totowa, NJ

strategy, the oligonucleotide is targeted to a specific sequence in the DNA double helix, thereby inhibiting gene transcription or permanently modifying the gene sequence. The main goal in the antigene strategy is to control in a sequence-specific manner the expression of a selected gene in a living cell. Because triplex-forming oligonucleotides (TFOs) bind specifically to duplex DNA, it has been proposed that triplex technology can serve as a foundation in the antigene strategy. Several reviews have appeared in the literature that describe a variety of approaches in which TFOs have been used *(1–4)*. In this chapter, we will focus on the use of TFOs in our research group to either target mutations to selected genes or promote recombination at selected sites in mammalian cells, thereby introducing permanent changes in the target sequence (Fig. 1).

2. TRIPLEX-FORMING OLIGONUCLEOTIDES

2.1. Binding Code

Triplex formation obeys precise rules imposed by several structural constraints *(5–7)*. TFOs bind in a sequence-specific manner via Hoogsteen binding as third strands in the major groove of duplex DNA. Triplex formation is favored at polypurine/polypyrimidine regions of DNA and can occur with the third strand oriented either parallel or antiparallel to the purine strand of the duplex. A TFO can be categorized according to its base composition and binding orientation relative to its DNA target site (Fig. 2). In the pyrimidine motif, a homopyrimidine TFO binds parallel to the purine strand of DNA via Hoogsteen bonds with the canonical triplets being T.A:T and C.G:C *(8,9)* (Fig. 2). Because protonation at the N3 position of cytosine is required for proper Hoogsteen binding with N7 guanine, pyrimidine oligonucleotides do not usually bind to DNA at physiological pH without further modification *(10)*. However, base modifications such as 5-methyl-2'-deoxycytidine can alleviate this pH dependence *(11,12)*. In the purine motif, a homopurine TFO binds antiparallel to the purine strand in the duplex via reverse Hoogsteen hydrogen bonds where the triplets are A.A:T and G.G:C *(5,13,14)* (Fig. 2). The ability of TFOs to bind tightly to DNA in a sequence-specific manner provides a powerful tool for genetic manipulation. Typically, for TFOs to have biological activity, they must bind with K_ds (dissociation constant) in the range of 10^{-9} *(15)*.

2.2. Stability

Although triplexes form more slowly than duplexes by several orders of magnitude, they are sufficiently stable to inhibit DNA-binding proteins once they are formed *(16–20)*. Several factors affect the binding affinity of TFOs. In addition to the sequence restriction of a polypurine site, several physiological conditions, including salt concentration and oligonucleotide length, contribute

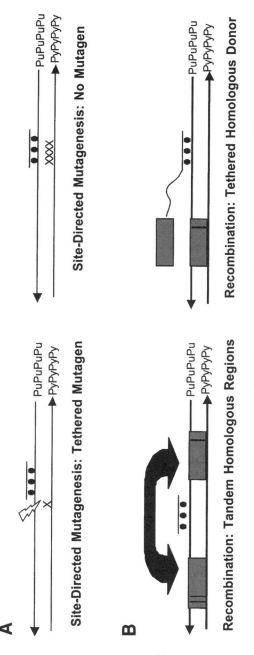

Fig. 1. Site-specific genome modification using triplex-forming oligonucleotides. (A) TFO-induced site-specific mutagenesis. (B) Gene conversion via homologous recombination.

29

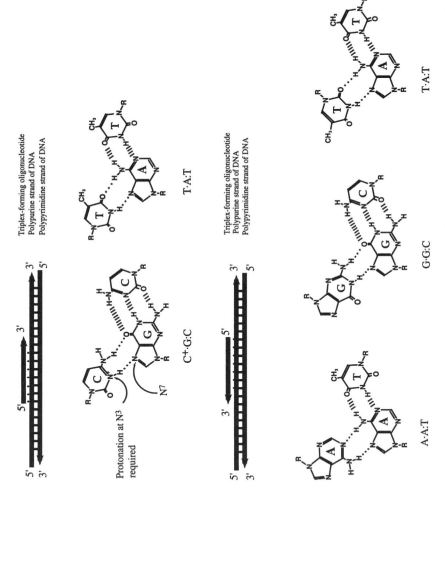

Fig. 2. Motifs for triple helix formation. (Top) In the pyrimidine motif, the third strand binds parallel to the purine strand of DNA via Hoogsteen bonds. (Bottom) In the purine motif, the third strand binds antiparallel to the purine strand via reverse Hoogsteen hydrogen bonds. The canonical base triplets are shown for each motif.

30

to binding affinity *(9,20)*. For instance, triplex formation is stabilized by divalent cations, such as magnesium and polyamines, which neutralize the charge repulsion between the negatively charged strands of the Watson–Crick duplex and the negatively charged backbone of the oligonucleotide *(21)*.

Although purine motif TFOs bind well at physiological pH, triplex formation via G-rich oligonucleotides can be inhibited by physiological concentrations of potassium *(22,23)*. This is a result of the formation of G-quartets and other secondary structures that appear to be stabilized by potassium *(24–26)*. Chemically modified bases, such as 7-deazaxanthine, can be used to help overcome the inhibitory effect of potassium *(27,28)*.

3. TARGETED MUTAGENESIS

Based on their sequence-specific binding and potential for molecular recognition of unique genomic sites, it was predicted that TFOs could be used to deliver a generally nonspecific mutagen to a specific site via intracellular triple helix formation *(29,30)*. Our laboratory and others have used a strategy in which the third strand was conjugated to the mutagen, psoralen, so that the sequence specificity of the TFO binding could induce site-specific DNA damage in a gene *(31–34)* (Fig. 1). Psoralen, a DNA intercalator, can covalently crosslink thymines on both strands of duplex DNA at 5' ApT 3' or 5' TpA 3' sites after photochemical activation using long wavelength ultraviolet A (UVA) irradiation. In earlier work, we tested the ability of a psoralen-linked TFO to induce site-specific mutations by targeting a polypurine/polypyrimidine run in the *supFG1* reporter gene in an SV40 vector *(29)*. The *supFG1* gene encodes an amber suppressor tyrosine tRNA and contains a 30-bp triplex target site. In bacteria with an amber mutation in the *lacZ* gene, a functional *supF* gene produces blue colonies on plates containing X-Gal and isopropyl-βD-thiogalactopyranoside (IPTG), whereas mutated versions produce white colonies. The frequency of mutagenesis is determined by the proportion of white colonies to blue colonies.

Using this approach, we have shown that psoralen-conjugated TFOs transfected into monkey COS cells can induce basepair-specific mutations within the *supFG1* mutation reporter gene in a SV40 genome in the cells, at frequencies in the range of 1–5% *(15)*. The key finding in this work was that the binding affinity of the TFO to its target site, as measured in vitro, was highly correlated with its intracellular activity. TFOs with K_ds (equilibrium dissociation constant) in the range of 10^{-9} M were more active; those with K_ds of 10^{-6} M were not.

3.1. TFO-Induced Mutagenesis at Chromosomal Sites

This work was extended to psoralen-TFO-mediated knockout of chromosomal genes. In one study, we used a mouse fibroblast cell line containing multiple copies of a λ *supFG1* shuttle vector DNA in a chromosomal locus *(35)*. The *supFG1* gene was again used as a target. The cells were treated by passive diffusion with the specific psoralen-conjugated TFO, psoAG30, or control TFO, psoSCR30, in the presence or absence of UVA irradiation *(35)*. After treatment, the replicated and repaired vector DNA was isolated from the mouse genomic DNA and packaged into phage particles using λ packaging extracts for subsequent mutational analysis *(36–38)*. Psoralen-conjugated AG30 induced mutations about 10-fold above background (psoSCR30-treated cells). This mutagenic effect was UVA-irradiation independent, demonstrating a mutagenesis process that is triplex mediated but photoproduct independent. Sequencing data further supports this result because the expected $T\bullet A \rightarrow A \bullet T$ transversions at the predicted psoralen crosslinking sites were not detected. However, insertions and deletions detected within the triplex binding site were consistent with a TFO-specific induction of mutagenesis *(35)*.

In the *supFG1* experiments, essentially unmodified G-rich oligonucleotides (except for 3' end capping) designed to bind in the anti-parallel motif were used. A set of experiments to target the hypoxanthine-guanine phosphoribosyl-transferase (*hprt*) gene in Chinese hamster ovary (CHO) fibroblasts *(39)*, in contrast, used a series of T-rich psoralen TFOs (because the A-rich target favored the parallel motif). In these experiments, the unmodified TFOs were ineffective. A second conjugation of the TFO to an intercalator, either acridine or pyrene, was needed to provide additional binding affinity. Such doubly modified TFOs yielded *hprt* mutagenesis at frequencies in the range of 10^{-4} to 10^{-3}, following electroporation of the TFOs into the cells, coupled with UVA irradiation to activate the psoralen.

However, the mutagenesis induced in the *supF* and *hprt* chromosomal targets, although site-specific in the sense that all the mutations clustered around the third-strand binding site, was somewhat variable. Hence, these experiments suggested that psoralen-coupled TFOs may be useful for gene-specific knockout but not necessarily for predictable basepair-specific mutagenesis. As a research tool, however, psoralen TFOs have served as useful reagents to prove the ability of oligonucleotides to bind as third strands to chromosomal sites in living cells. The importance of this result is to establish the concept that DNA-binding molecules can be used to direct site-specific genome modification and to show that the cell and nuclear membranes and the packaging of the DNA into chromatin are not absolute barriers to gene targeting with antigene oligonucleotides.

In the course of this work with psoralen TFOs, we observed that unconjugated TFOs were also capable of inducing mutations in the target gene, at least when the binding affinity was sufficiently high *(40)* (Fig. 1). The effect was shown to be a consequence of the stimulation of DNA repair by the formation of a triple helix, which seems to be recognized by the nucleotide excision repair (NER) complex as a "lesion" *(40)*. No mutagenesis was detected above background in the *supFG1* gene in cell lines deficient in NER (xeroderma pigmentosum group

A [XPA] cells) or in transcription-coupled repair (TCR) (Cockayne's syndrome B [CSB] cells) after treatment with unconjugated TFOs *(40)*. In addition, triplex formation was found to stimulate DNA repair synthesis in human cell-free extracts.

Although this work provided indirect evidence of the requirement of NER machinery in the triplex-directed mutagenic pathway, the mechanism for triplex recognition remained unknown. Studies designed to determine the roles of XPA and replication protein A (RPA) in the recognition of triple helices were performed *(41)*. We obtained direct evidence for recognition of triplexes by the human XPA–RPA repair complex, leading to DNA repair activity that generates recombination intermediates. RPA binds to triplex DNA with high affinity, with or without XPA, whereas XPA binds only in conjunction with RPA *(41)*. However, XPA contributes to specificity by selectively diminishing nonspecific binding of RPA to undamaged DNA.

Recently, Vasquez *(42)* demonstrated that TFOs are capable of inducing specific mutations in the somatic cells of adult mice. Transgenic mice (3340), bearing multiple copies of a chromosomally integrated λ supFG1 vector, which contains the *supFG1* reporter gene with the 30-basepair triplex target site, were used in this study (Fig. 3). The mice were treated intraperitoneally for 5 consecutive days with either AG30 or the nonspecific control oligonucleotide, SCR30. Ten days post-treatment, the mice were sacrificed and their tissues collected for mutational analysis. The combined mutation frequency in a variety of tissues from mice treated with AG30 (27×10^{-5}) increased by about fivefold in comparison to the tissues from SCR30-treated mice (5.4×10^{-5}). All tissues tested exhibited TFO-induced mutagenesis, except for the brain, which had no mutations above background. This result is consistent with the fact that oligonucleotides do not efficiently cross the blood–brain barrier after intraperitoneal injection *(43)*. The level of mutagenesis observed in tissues of mice treated with SCR30 did not differ significantly from those treated with PBS. Therefore, nonspecific oligonucleotides do not appear to be mutagenic. Additionally, the effects of AG30 are target site-specific as nearly 85% of the mutations in the *supF* gene were clustered within the triplex target site *(42)*, and no induction of mutagenesis above background was observed in another mutation reporter gene, *cII*. Thus, it is apparent given these results that gene modification via triplex formation is a possible approach to gene knockout in animals.

4. TARGETED RECOMBINATION

Homologous recombination provides another gene therapy strategy that can be used to modify the genome for the purpose of gene replacement or gene correction *(1)*. However, this technique is limited by low efficiency of homologous integration (10^{-8} to 10^{-9} homologous events per cell), and a high rate of

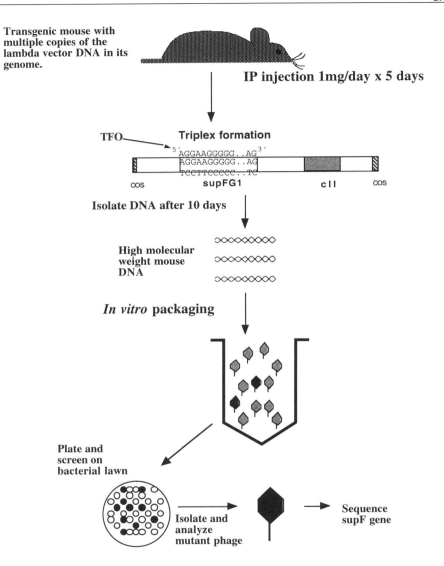

Fig. 3. Experimental protocol for detecting chromosomal mutations after administration of TFOs in mice. Adult transgenic mice containing multiple copies of chromosomally integrated λ supFG1 vector, which contains the 30 bp triplex target site, were injected intraperitoneally with TFOs. Following treatment, tissues were collected, and genomic DNA was isolated and analyzed. In vitro packaging of the phage vector led to detection of mutagenesis via plating on a bacterial lawn. If no mutations occur in the *supFG1* gene, the plaques will appear blue in the presence of IPTG and X-Gal. However, if a mutation does occur, the resulting plaques will be white.

random integrations of the vector DNA. Investigators have recognized that the ability to sensitize a target site to homologous recombination may potentially enhance the frequency of homologous integration in mammalian cells *(44)*. It has been demonstrated that DNA damage, such as double-strand breaks, can stimulate homologous recombination *(45)*. However, although DNA-damaging agents may enhance recombinogenic events, they do not address the issue of nonspecific homologous integration and therefore can not be used for gene-targeting purposes *(46–48)*. Site-specific triplex formation represents one potential tool for stimulation of a target site to recombination. Based on the concept that third-strand binding, with or without psoralen coupling, can trigger DNA repair, we hypothesized that triplexes could sensitize a target site to homologous recombination by the same mechanism.

4.1. Induced Recombination Between Two Mutant Genes

Using an SV40 vector containing two mutant copies of the *supF* gene as tandem repeats, we found that both psoralen TFOs *(49)* and unconjugated TFOs *(50)* can trigger recombination within an SV40 virus genome (Fig. 4). Each of the *supF* genes contained a single inactivating point mutation but at different position in the gene. Additionally, the upstream *supF1* gene contained at the 3' end the 30-basepair polypurine high-affinity triplex-binding sequence (Fig. 4A). Thus, targeted damage at the triplex-binding site could potentially induce recombination between the two mutant *supF* genes to produce a fully functional *supF* gene, which could be identified in our assay as blue colonies on indicator plates. The psoralen TFO-stimulated recombination to generate a wild-type *supF* gene at a frequency of 1.5%, nearly 25-fold above background *(50)*. When unconjugated TFOs were used, recombinants were generated at a frequency of 0.37%, approximately fivefold above background. The induced recombination in the absence of psoralen was found to be dependent on the presence of functional XPA protein *(50)*. However, recombination induced by psoralen triplexes was only partially dependent on NER. In XPA-deficient cells, psoralen TFOs still stimulated recombination to a substantial degree.

Our laboratory extended these results to a chromosomal target by constructing a mouse LTK⁻ cell line with two mutant copies of the herpes simplex virus thymidine kinase (TK) gene as direct repeats in a single chromosomal site (Fig. 4B). A third-strand-binding site was situated between the two genes. Transfection (via cationic lipids) of cells with high-affinity TFOs targeting the region between the two genes yielded recombination at a frequency of approximately sevenfold above background *(51)*. When the TFOs were micro-injected into the nuclei of the cells (~70,000 copies/cell), the yield of recombinants increased to 1–2%, 3000-fold over background. Analysis of the recombinant clones revealed that all the recombination events involved gene conversion rather than crossover recombination. In addition to establishing the capability to induce recombination

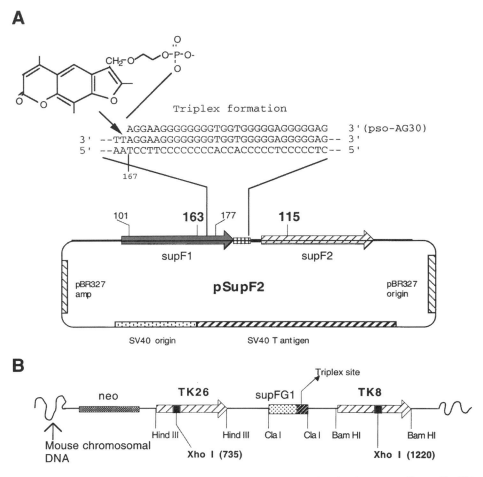

Fig. 4. Vectors used in the detection of triplex-induced recombination in mammalian cells. (**A**) SV40 shuttle vector containing two mutant copies of the *supF* gene. (**B**) Chromosomal target in mouse cells with two mutant copies of the herpes simplex virus thymidine kinase (TK) gene in tandem repeat.

at a chromosomal target, these experiments revealed the importance of intra-nuclear delivery to achieve sufficient levels of targeted genome modification.

4.2. Induced Recombination Using a TFO Tethered to a Donor Fragment

Our observation that third-strand binding can provoke DNA repair and stimu-late recombination led us to develop a strategy to mediate targeted gene conver-sion using a bifunctional oligonucleotide composed of a TFO coupled to a short donor fragment homologous to the target gene (except at the basepair to be corrected) *(52)*. In this tethered-donor strategy, the TFO domain is intended to bind to the gene, thereby positioning the donor fragment for recombination and information transfer (Fig. 1). Additionally, the formation of a triple helix can trigger repair, thereby sensitizing the target site to recombination. The tethered homologous donor fragment can then participate in recombination and/or gene conversion with the target gene to correct or alter the nucleotide sequence.

Such a bifunctional oligomer, A-AG30, consisting of a 40-mer donor domain and a 30-mer TFO domain, was found to mediate correction of a single point mutation in the extrachromosomal *supFG1* reporter gene within an SV40 vector in monkey COS cells in culture. The target vector, pSupFG1/G144C, contained a mutated version of the *supFG1* amber suppressor tRNA gene, *supFG1-144*, which has an inactivating G:C to C:G mutation at bp 144. In the tethered-donor molecule, A-AG30, the donor fragment A consists of a single-strand, 40 nucleotides in length, synthesized to be homologous to positions 121–160 of the *supFG1-144* gene, except at position 144, where the sequence matches that of the functional *supFG1* gene. Correction frequencies were in the range of 0.1% with the full bifunctional molecule. Oligomers consisting of either domain alone or either domain substituted with control sequences reduced activity by 10-fold or more. The donor domain alone consistently did mediate some gene correction, as would be expected, based on the known ability of DNA fragments to mediate some level of recombination. However, there was a clear synergism to combination with the TFO domain.

To elucidate the mechanism by which triplexes induce recombination, we also examined the ability of the bifunctional molecule, A-AG30, to induce recombination in human cell-free extracts. An assay for reversion of a point mutation in the *supFG1* gene in the plasmid pSupFG1/G144C was established in which recombination in extracts was detected upon transformation into indicator bacteria. The oligomer was incubated with the target vector in HeLa cell-free extracts supplemented with an ATP regenerating system. After a 2-h incubation period and isolation of the plasmid vector DNA, the oligomer was found to mediate gene correction in vitro at a frequency of 46×10^{-5}, 20-fold above background and fourfold greater than donor alone *(53)*. This effect was determined to occur in the extracts and not in the indicator bacteria because no recombinants were observed unless the samples had been incubated in the extracts. Interestingly, physical linkage of the TFO to the donor was not necessary, as comixture of the two segments resulted in an elevated gene correction frequency of 40×10^{-5}, almost as high as that produced by the linked oligomer. This demonstrates that the role of the TFO in stimulating recombination is distinct from its ability to position the donor fragment for information transfer at the target site. Upon immunodepletion of the repair and recombination proteins, XPA and HsRad51, triplex-induced recombination was diminished. However, supplementation of the purified proteins resulted in partial or complete restoration of activity. These results demonstrate that triplex-induced recombination is dependent on NER and homologous recombinational repair of NER-generated intermediates.

5. PEPTIDE NUCLEIC ACIDS

Another class of DNA-binding reagents that can be used in genome modification are peptide nucleic acids (PNAs). PNA is a DNA mimic in which the purine and pyrimidine bases are attached to a polyamide backbone rather than the normal phosphodiester backbone. This backbone maintains a spacing similar to DNA, but yields an achiral, neutrally charged molecule. Additionally, PNAs are resistant to cellular nucleases and proteases. PNAs can bind to DNA via Watson–Crick hydrogen bonds, with binding affinities significantly higher than those of the corresponding DNA oligomers *(54)*. It has been shown that PNAs can bind to complementary sequences in duplex DNA by strand invasion. This results in the displacement of one DNA strand and the formation of a D-loop *(55)*. Highly stable PNA:DNA:PNA triplexes are formed when two PNA molecules are available to bind to one DNA strand or two strands of PNA are connected by a flexible linker (PNA clamp). In this structure, one strand forms Watson–Crick basepairs with the displaced strand in an antiparallel orientation, whereas the other strand forms Hoogsteen basepairs to the DNA–PNA duplex *(56)*. Because even moderate concentrations of cations can stabilize duplex DNA, thereby reducing accessibility for strand invasion, the binding efficiency of PNA may be severely decreased in vivo. However, it has been found that the transcription process, by either transiently opening the DNA double helix in the transcription bubble or indirectly creating local negative DNA super-helical tension, may dramatically improve PNA binding under physiological conditions *(57,58)*. PNA triplex strand invasion complexes are sufficiently stable to arrest transcription initiation and elongation *(59)*. Additionally, PNAs can inhibit binding of proteins, such as restriction enzymes and transcriptional factors, to their target site *(60)*.

5.1. Site-Specific Mutagenesis Induced by PNA

Because high-affinity triplex formation has been shown to provoke site-specific mutagenesis, we designed a bis-PNA to bind as a clamp to a site in the *supFG1* mutation reporter gene, to determine whether PNA binding might also induce mutagenesis *(61)*. Transgenic mouse fibroblasts, with multiple chromosomally integrated copies of recoverable λ phage shuttle vector carrying the *supFG1* reporter gene, were permeabilized with streptolysin-*O*. Efficient cellular uptake of the PNA was detected through the use of confocal microscopy and fluorescein-conjugated PNAs. Phage vector rescue and reporter gene analysis revealed that the PNA-induced mutations in *supFG1* at a frequency of 0.1% (10-fold above background) *(61)*. No increased mutagenesis was detected in the nontargeted *cII* gene, indicating the specificity of the PNA-induced mutagenesis. Sequence analysis revealed that the majority of mutants were located within the PNA-binding site and consisted mostly of insertion and deletions. This suggests that the high-affinity binding PNA clamp may provoke replication slippage errors. The ability of a PNA clamp to induce mutations and provoke DNA metabolism may prove useful as a tool in gene therapy.

6. LIMITATIONS AND FUTURE CHALLENGES

Although triplex technology is quite promising, it does suffer from important constraints, including inefficient delivery and restrictions on permitted target sequences. Cellular uptake, intracellular compartmentalization, and bioavailability need to be improved to increase the efficacy of TFOs. To induce permanent genomic modification, the compounds must reach the target DNA located in the nucleus. Unfortunately, most data suggest that oligonucleotides are taken up by endocytosis and therefore might be trapped in endocytic vesicles within the cytoplasm. Experiments in which oligonucleotides have been microinjected directly into the nucleus show a great enhancement in their efficacy *(51)*. As a result, one can conclude that delivery must play an important role in determining the biological activity of an oligonucleotide. Numerous strategies have been explored to enhance oligonucleotide delivery, including cationic lipids *(62,63)*, cell permeabilization reagents such as digitonin *(49,64,65)*, and square wave electroporation *(66)*. Additionally, peptide conjugates have been used to improve both intracellular uptake and compartmentalization. Three peptides that have been used to increase intracellular distribution of oligonucleotides are transportan *(67)*, Antennapedia *(68)*, and TAT *(69)*. These carrier peptides exhibit different preferences in their intracellular localization.

Although the data discussed here have implicated pathways by which TFOs induce recombination and mutagenesis, the exact mechanisms still remain unknown. Thus, studies that establish the precise cellular processes involved in genomic modifications are necessary. Additionally, it is important to determine which factors, such as transcription levels, cell-cycle phase, nucleosome binding and histone state, play a role in the availability of genomic targets to DNA-binding compounds.

Because of the low correction frequencies obtained with TFO usage, triplex technology may not be applicable to all disease types, particularly those that require large populations of cells to be corrected. Instead, this technology may be applied to certain hematologic diseases, such as sickle-cell anemia, in which only a small percentage of correction may be required for amelioration of the disease state. Nonetheless, although triplex technology is faced with some limitations, it still remains a potentially powerful tool for genomic modification. Further advances in this area may eventually enable its therapeutic potential to be realized.

REFERENCES

1. Vasquez KM, Wilson JH. Triplex-directed modification of genes and gene activity. Trends Biochem Sci 1998; 23:4–9.
2. Praseuth D, Guieysse AL, Helene C. Triple helix formation and the antigene strategy for sequence-specific control of gene expression. Biochim Biophys Acta 1999; 1489:181–206.
3. Chan PP, Glazer PM. Triplex DNA: fundamentals, advances, and potential applications for gene therapy. J Mol Med 1997; 75:267–82.
4. Curcio LD, Bouffard DY, Scanlon KJ. Oligonucleotides as modulators of cancer gene expression. Pharmacol Ther 1997; 74:317–32.
5. Letai AG, Palladino MA, Fromm E, Rizzo V, Fresco JR. Specificity in formation of triple-stranded nucleic acid helical complexes: studies with agarose-linked polyribonucleotide affinity columns. Biochemistry 1988; 27:9108–12.
6. Francois JC, Saison-Behmoaras T, Helene C. Sequence-specific recognition of the major groove of DNA by oligodeoxynucleotides via triple helix formation. Footprinting studies. Nucleic Acids Res 1988; 16:11431–40.
7. Cooney M, Czernuszewicz G, Postel EH, Flint SJ, Hogan ME. Site-specific oligonucleotide binding represses transcription of the human c-myc gene in vitro. Science 1988; 241:456–9.
8. Le Doan T, Perrouault L, Praseuth D, et al. Sequence-specific recognition, photocrosslinking and cleavage of the DNA double helix by an oligo-[alpha]-thymidylate covalently linked to an azidoproflavine derivative. Nucleic Acids Res 1987; 15:7749–60.
9. Moser HE, Dervan PB. Sequence-specific cleavage of double helical DNA by triple helix formation. Science 1987; 238:645–50.
10. Lee JS, Johnson DA, Morgan AR. Complexes formed by (pyrimidine)n . (purine)n DNAs on lowering the pH are three-stranded. Nucleic Acids Res 1979; 6:3073–91.
11. Povsic TJ, Dervan PB. Triple helix formation by oligonucleotides on DNA extended to the physiological range. J Am Chem Soc 1989; 111:3059–3061.
12. Lacroix L, Lacoste J, Reddoch JF, et al. Triplex formation by oligonucleotides containing 5-(1-propynyl)-2'-deoxyuridine: decreased magnesium dependence and improved intracellular gene targeting. Biochemistry 1999; 38:1893–901.
13. Beal PA, Dervan PB. Second structural motif for recognition of DNA by oligonucleotide-directed triple-helix formation. Science 1991; 251:1360–3.
14. Durland RH, Kessler DJ, Gunnell S, Duvic M, Pettitt BM, Hogan ME. Binding of triple helix forming oligonucleotides to sites in gene promoters. Biochemistry 1991; 30:9246–55.
15. Wang G, Levy DD, Seidman MM, Glazer PM. Targeted mutagenesis in mammalian cells mediated by intracellular triple helix formation. Mol Cell Biol 1995; 15:1759–68.
16. Maher LJ, Wold B, Dervan PB. Inhibition of DNA binding proteins by oligonucleotide-directed triple helix formation. Science 1989; 245:725–30.
17. Maher LJ, Dervan PB, Wold BJ. Kinetic analysis of oligodeoxyribonucleotide-directed triple-helix formation on DNA. Biochemistry 1990; 29:8820–6.
18. Musso M, Wang JC, Van Dyke MW. In vivo persistence of DNA triple helices containing psoralen-conjugated oligodeoxyribonucleotides. Nucleic Acids Res 1996; 24:4924–32.
19. Svinarchuk F, Debin A, Bertrand JR, Malvy C. Investigation of the intracellular stability and formation of a triple helix formed with a short purine oligonucleotide targeted to the murine c-pim-1 proto-oncogene promotor. Nucleic Acids Res 1996; 24:295–302.
20. Rougee M, Faucon B, Mergny JL, et al. Kinetics and thermodynamics of triple-helix formation: effects of ionic strength and mismatches. Biochemistry 1992; 31:9269–78.
21. Hampel KJ, Crosson P, Lee JS. Polyamines favor DNA triplex formation at neutral pH. Biochemistry 1991; 30:4455–9.
22. Cheng AJ, Van Dyke MW. Monovalent cation effects on intermolecular purine-purine-pyrimidine triple-helix formation. Nucleic Acids Res 1993; 21:5630–5.

23. Olivas WM, Maher LJ. Overcoming potassium-mediated triplex inhibition. Nucleic Acids Res 1995; 23:1936–41.
24. Olivas WM, Maher LJ. Competitive triplex/quadruplex equilibria involving guanine-rich oligonucleotides. Biochemistry 1995; 34:278–84.
25. Sen D, Gilbert W. A sodium-potassium switch in the formation of four-stranded G4-DNA. Nature 1990; 344:410–414.
26. Williamson JR, Raghuraman MK, Cech TR. Monovalent cation-induced structure of telomeric DNA: the G-quartet model. Cell 1989; 59:871–880.
27. Milligan JF, Krawczyk SH, Wadwani S, Matteucci MD. An anti-parallel triple helix motif with oligodeoxynucleotides containing 2'-deoxyguanosine and 7-deaza-2'-deoxyxanthosine. Nucleic Acids Res 1993; 21:327–33.
28. Faruqi AF, Krawczyk SH, Matteucci MD, Glazer PM. Potassium-resistant triple helix formation and improved intracellular gene targeting by oligodeoxyribonucleotides containing 7-deazaxanthine. Nucleic Acids Res 1997; 25:633–40.
29. Havre PA, Gunther EJ, Gasparro FP, Glazer PM. Targeted mutagenesis of DNA using triple helix-forming oligonucleotides linked to psoralen. Proc Natl Acad Sci USA 1993; 90:7879–83.
30. Havre PA, Glazer PM. Targeted mutagenesis of simian virus 40 DNA mediated by a triple helix-forming oligonucleotide. J Virol 1993; 67:7324–31.
31. Sandor Z, Bredberg A. Repair of triple helix directed psoralen adducts in human cells. Nucleic Acids Res 1994; 22:2051–6.
32. Gasparro FP, Havre PA, Olack GA, Gunther EJ, Glazer PM. Site-specific targeting of psoralen photoadducts with a triple helix-forming oligonucleotide: characterization of psoralen monoadduct and crosslink formation. Nucleic Acids Res 1994; 22:2845–52.
33. Takasugi M, Guendouz A, Chassignol M, et al. Sequence-specific photo-induced cross-linking of the two strands of double-helical DNA by a psoralen covalently linked to a triple helix-forming oligonucleotide. Proc Natl Acad Sci USA 1991; 88:5602–6.
34. Giovannangeli C, Thuong NT, Helene C. Oligodeoxynucleotide-directed photo-induced cross-linking of HIV proviral DNA via triple-helix formation. Nucleic Acids Res 1992; 20:4275–81.
35. Vasquez KM, Wang G, Havre PA, Glazer PM. Chromosomal mutations induced by triplex-forming oligonucleotides in mammalian cells. Nucleic Acids Res 1999; 27:1176–81.
36. Glazer PM, Sarkar SN, Summers WC. Detection and analysis of UV-induced mutations in mammalian cell DNA using a lambda phage shuttle vector. Proc Natl Acad Sci USA 1986; 83:1041–4.
37. Gunther EJ, Murray NE, Glazer PM. High efficiency, restriction-deficient in vitro packaging extracts for bacteriophage lambda DNA using a new E.coli lysogen. Nucleic Acids Res 1993; 21:3903–4.
38. Narayanan L, Fritzell JA, Baker SM, Liskay RM, Glazer PM. Elevated levels of mutation in multiple tissues of mice deficient in the DNA mismatch repair gene Pms2. Proc Natl Acad Sci USA 1997; 94:3122–7.
39. Majumdar A, Khorlin A, Dyatkina N, et al. Targeted gene knockout mediated by triple helix forming oligonucleotides. Nat Genet 1998; 20:212–4.
40. Wang G, Seidman MM, Glazer PM. Mutagenesis in mammalian cells induced by triple helix formation and transcription-coupled repair. Science 1996; 271:802–5.
41. Vasquez KM, Christensen J, Li L, Finch RA, Glazer PM. Human XPA and RPA DNA repair proteins participate in specific recognition of triplex-induced helical distortions. Proc Natl Acad Sci USA 2002; 99:5848–53.
42. Vasquez KM, Narayanan L, Glazer PM. Specific mutations induced by triplex-forming oligonucleotides in mice. Science 2000; 290:530–3.
43. Zendegui JG, Vasquez KM, Tinsley JH, Kessler DJ, Hogan ME. In vivo stability and kinetics of absorption and disposition of 3' phosphopropyl amine oligonucleotides. Nucleic Acids Res 1992; 20:307–14.

44. Vasquez KM, Marburger K, Intody Z, Wilson JH. Manipulating the mammalian genome by homologous recombination. Proc Natl Acad Sci USA 2001; 98:8403–10.
45. Rouet P, Smih F, Jasin M. Introduction of double-strand breaks into the genome of mouse cells by expression of a rare-cutting endonuclease. Mol Cell Biol 1994; 14:8096–106.
46. Saffran WA, Cantor CR, Smith ED, Magdi M. Psoralen damage-induced plasmid recombination in Saccharomyces cerevisiae: dependence on RAD1 and RAD52. Mutat Res 1992; 274:1–9.
47. Wang YY, Maher VM, Liskay RM, McCormick JJ. Carcinogens can induce homologous recombination between duplicated chromosomal sequences in mouse L cells. Mol Cell Biol 1988; 8:196–202.
48. Tsujimura T, Maher VM, Godwin AR, Liskay RM, McCormick JJ. Frequency of intra-chromosomal homologous recombination induced by UV radiation in normally repairing and excision repair-deficient human cells. Proc Natl Acad Sci USA 1990; 87:1566–70.
49. Faruqi AF, Seidman MM, Segal DJ, Carroll D, Glazer PM. Recombination induced by triple-helix-targeted DNA damage in mammalian cells. Mol Cell Biol 1996; 16:6820–8.
50. Faruqi AF, Datta HJ, Carroll D, Seidman MM, Glazer PM. Triple-helix formation induces recombination in mammalian cells via a nucleotide excision repair-dependent pathway. Mol Cell Biol 2000; 20:990–1000.
51. Luo Z, Macris MA, Faruqi AF, Glazer PM. High-frequency intrachromosomal gene conversion induced by triplex-forming oligonucleotides microinjected into mouse cells. Proc Natl Acad Sci USA 2000; 97:9003–8.
52. Chan PP, Lin M, Faruqi AF, Powell J, Seidman MM, Glazer PM. Targeted correction of an episomal gene in mammalian cells by a short DNA fragment tethered to a triplex-forming oligonucleotide. J Biol Chem 1999; 274:11541–8.
53. Datta HJ, Chan PP, Vasquez KM, Gupta RC, Glazer PM. Triplex-induced recombination in human cell-free extracts. Dependence on XPA and HsRad51. J Biol Chem 2001; 276:18018–23.
54. Egholm M, Buchardt O, Christensen L, et al. PNA hybridizes to complementary oligonucleotides obeying the Watson-Crick hydrogen-bonding rules. Nature 1993; 365:566–8.
55. Peffer NJ, Hanvey JC, Bisi JE, et al. Strand-invasion of duplex DNA by peptide nucleic acid oligomers. Proc Natl Acad Sci USA 1993; 90:10648–52.
56. Egholm M, Christensen L, Dueholm KL, Buchardt O, Coull J, Nielsen PE. Efficient pH-independent sequence-specific DNA binding by pseudoisocytosine-containing bis-PNA. Nucleic Acids Res 1995; 23:217–22.
57. Larsen HJ, Nielsen PE. Transcription-mediated binding of peptide nucleic acid (PNA) to double-stranded DNA: sequence-specific suicide transcription. Nucleic Acids Res 1996; 24:458–63.
58. Bentin T, Nielsen PE. Enhanced peptide nucleic acid binding to supercoiled DNA: possible implications for DNA "breathing" dynamics. Biochemistry 1996; 35:8863–9.
59. Praseuth D, Grigoriev M, Guieysse AL, et al. Peptide nucleic acids directed to the promoter of the alpha-chain of the interleukin-2 receptor. Biochim Biophys Acta 1996; 1309:226–38.
60. Nielsen PE, Egholm M, Berg RH, Buchardt O. Sequence specific inhibition of DNA restriction enzyme cleavage by PNA. Nucleic Acids Res 1993; 21:197–200.
61. Faruqi AF, Egholm M, Glazer PM. Peptide nucleic acid-targeted mutagenesis of a chromosomal gene in mouse cells. Proc Natl Acad Sci USA 1998; 95:1398–403.
62. Hobbs CA, Yoon K. Differential regulation of gene expression in vivo by triple helix-forming oligonucleotides as detected by a reporter enzyme. Antisense Res Dev 1994; 4:1–8.
63. Porumb H, Gousset H, Letellier R, et al. Temporary ex vivo inhibition of the expression of the human oncogene HER2 (NEU) by a triple helix-forming oligonucleotide. Cancer Res 1996; 56:515–22.
64. Macaulay VM, Bates PJ, McLean MJ, et al. Inhibition of aromatase expression by a psoralen-linked triplex-forming oligonucleotide targeted to a coding sequence. FEBS Lett 1995; 372:222–8.

65. Kochetkova M, Shannon MF. DNA triplex formation selectively inhibits granulocyte-macrophage colony-stimulating factor gene expression in human T cells. J Biol Chem 1996; 271:14438–44.
66. Liu Y, Began R. Improved Intracellular Delivery of Oligonucleotides by Square Wave Electroporation. Antisense & Nucleic Acid Drug Development 2001; 11:7–14.
67. Pooga M, Hallbrink M, Zorko M, Langel U. Cell penetration by transportan. Faseb J 1998; 12:67–77.
68. Derossi D, Joliot AH, Chassaing G, Prochiantz A. The third helix of the Antennapedia homeodomain translocates through biological membranes. J Biol Chem 1994; 269:10444–50.
69. Tung CH, Wang J, Leibowitz MJ, Stein S. Dual-specificity interaction of HIV-1 TAR RNA with tat peptide-oligonucleotide conjugates. Bioconjug Chem 1995; 6:292–5.

4 Therapeutic Applications of Ribozymes

John J. Rossi, PhD

1. INTRODUCTION

Ribozymes are RNA molecules capable of acting as enzymes even in the complete absence of proteins. They have the catalytic activity of breaking and/or forming covalent bonds with extraordinary specificity, accelerating the rate of these reactions. The ability of RNA to serve as a catalyst was first shown for the self-splicing Group I intron of *Tetrahymena* and the RNA moiety of RNase P *(1–3)*. Subsequent to the discovery of these two RNA enzymes, RNA-mediated catalysis has been found associated with the self-splicing group II introns of yeast, fungal and plant mitochondria (as well as chloroplasts) *(4)*, single-stranded plant viroid and virusoid RNAs *(5–7)*, hepatitis delta virus *(8)*, and a satellite RNA from *Neurospora* mitochondria *(9)*. It is rather clear that the RNA component of the larger ribosomal subunit is functioning as a peptidyltransferase as

From: *Cancer Drug Discovery and Development:*
Nucleic Acid Therapeutics in Cancer
Edited by: A. M. Gewirtz © Humana Press Inc., Totowa, NJ

well *(10–12)*. The potential functioning of spliceosomal snRNAs as a ribozyme in complex with the pre-mRNA to catalyze pre-messenger-RNA splicing has also been proposed *(13)*. It is highly likely that additional RNA catalytic motifs and new roles for RNA-mediated catalysis will also be found as we learn more about the genomes of a variety of organisms.

Ribozymes occur naturally but can also be artificially engineered and synthesized to target-specific sequences in *cis* or *trans*. New biochemical activities are being developed using in vitro selection protocols as well *(14)*. Ribozymes can easily be manipulated to act on novel substrates. These custom-designed RNAs have great potential as therapeutic agents and are becoming a powerful tool for molecular biologists.

The discovery of catalytic RNA molecules has revolutionized views on the origins of life. RNA molecules, once thought to be primarily passive carriers of genetic information, can carry out some functions previously only thought to be catalyzed by proteins, indicating that RNA can confer not only a genotype (as in many RNA viruses) but also a phenotype. The RNA-catalyzed reactions include self-cleavage, or *trans* cleavage reactions, ligation, and *trans*-splicing. These observations have led to speculation that RNA might have been an early self-replicating molecule in the prebiotic world. Evidence supporting this notion comes from the fact that group I introns can exhibit RNA-polymerase-like activities under certain conditions *(15)*. In addition, the catalytic core of group I introns shares homology with several small satellite RNAs associated with plant viruses, which are also homologous to the human hepatitis delta virus (HDV), suggesting a common and ancient origin.

2. CATALYTIC MOTIFS

There are six ribozymes that have been successfully modified or adapted for use in therapeutic and functional genomic applications. These are the group I introns, RNase P, the hammerhead and hairpin motifs, the hepatitis delta ribozyme, and the reverse-splicing reaction of group II introns. Each of the above ribozymes requires a divalent metal cation for activity (usually Mg++), which may participate in the chemistry of the cleavage or ligation reaction or may be important for maintaining the structure of the ribozyme.

The group I intron of *Tetrahymena* was the first ribozyme for which the *cis*-cleaving (on a portion of the same RNA strand) reaction was converted into a *trans*- (on an exogenous RNA molecule) reaction *(2)*. An altered form of the ribozyme lacking the 5' and 3' exons, but with a guanosine covalently attached to the 3' end of the intron, was shown to be capable of binding RNA substrates with complementarity to an internal guide sequence, cleaving the bound RNA, releasing the cleavage products, and recycling the ribozyme itself. A more recent application of the group I intron is that of correcting defective mRNAs in what has been termed *"trans*-splicing" *(16)*. In its *trans*-splicing configuration, the group I intron is not attached to a 5' exon, but has appended to the intron a 3' exon, which is to be *trans*-spliced onto a target RNA. *Trans*-splicing may be of clinical importance in the future for repairing defective messages *(17)*.

The group II intron was first identified as a self-splicing ribozyme in fungal mitochondrial transcripts. Since the initial discovery, these introns have been found in chloroplasts as well as in some bacteria *(4)*. The intron has two sequences called "exon binding sites" (EBS), which pair with sequences in the exons during self-splicing. The released intron can reinsert itself into spliced RNA, as well as DNA, by a reversal of the splicing mechanism. The sequence requirements for binding of the EBS elements to a target DNA have been elucidated, allowing engineering of the EBS for targeted integration of the group II introns into a variety of gene sequences *(18)*. The implications of this work are that group II introns can be engineered for targeted gene disruption or for insertion of thera-peutic genes in a site-specific fashion into a host genome.

The endoribonuclease RNase P is found in organisms throughout nature. As stated previously, this enzyme has RNA and one or more protein components. The RNA component from the *E. coli* and *B. subtilis* enzymes can act as a site-specific cleavage agent in the absence of the protein under certain salt and ionic conditions *(19)*. Studies of the substrate requirements for this enzyme isolated from either bacteria or humans have been carried out. The minimal substrates for either the bacterial or human enzymes resemble a segment of a transfer RNA molecule *(20,21)*. This structure can be mimicked by uniquely designed antisense RNAs, which pair to the target RNA, and serve as substrates for RNase P medi-ated site-specific cleavage. It has also been shown that the antisense component can be covalently joined to the RNase P RNA, thereby directing the enzyme only to the target RNA of interest *(22)*. Investigators have taken advantage of this property in the design of antisense RNAs, which pair with target mRNAs of interest, to stimulate site-specific cleavage of the target and recycling of the antisense *(23–26)*.

One category of intramolecular RNA catalysis is that which produces a 2', 3'-cyclic phosphate and 5'-OH terminus on the reaction products. A number of small plant-pathogenic RNAs (viroids, satellite RNAs, and virusoids), a tran-script from a *Neurospora* mitochondrial DNA plasmid, and the animal virus HDV undergo a self-cleavage reaction in vitro in the absence of protein. The reactions require neutral pH and Mg^{2+}. It is thought that the self-cleavage reac-tion is an integral part of their in vivo rolling circle mechanism of replication. These self-cleaving RNAs can be subdivided into groups according to the se-quence and secondary structure formed about the cleavage site. Small ribozymes have been derived from a motif found in single-stranded plant viroid and virusoid RNAs that replicate via a rolling circle mechanism. Based on a shared secondary structure and a conserved set of nucleotides, the term *hammerhead* has been given to one group of this self-cleavage domain *(27,28)*. The hammerhead ribozyme is composed of approx 30 nucleotides. The simplicity of the hammerhead catalytic domain (Fig. 1) has made it a popular choice in the design of *trans*-acting ribozymes. Utilizing Watson–Crick basepairing, the hammerhead ribozyme can be designed to cleave any target RNA. The requirements at the cleavage site are relatively simple, and virtually any UH (where H is U, C, or A) can be targeted.

A second plant-derived self-cleavage motif, initially identified in the negative strand of the tobacco ringspot satellite RNA, has been termed the "hairpin" or "paperclip" (Fig. 1) *(7)*. The hairpin ribozymes cleave RNA substrates in a reversible reaction that generates 2', 3'-cyclic phosphate and 5'-hydroxyl termini. Engineered versions of this catalytic motif have also been shown to be capable of cleaving and turning over multiple copies of a variety of targets in *trans* (Fig. 2)*(29)*. Substrate requirements for the hairpin include a GUC, with cleavage occurring immediately upstream of the G. The hairpin ribozyme is also capable of catalyzing a ligation reaction, although it is more frequently used for cleavage reactions. Hairpin ribozyme-mediated cleavage and ligation proceed through a catalytic mechanism that does not require direct coordination of metal cations to phosphate or water oxygens.

The HDV genomic and antigenomic RNAs contain a self-cleavage site hypothesized to function during rolling circle replication of this satellite virus. Like the plant pathogens, the sites in HDV are postulated to have a related secondary structure, three models of which have been proposed: *cloverleaf*, *pseudoknot*, and *axehead (30)*, none of which is similar to the catalytic domains previously described. Like the other ribozyme motifs, the HDV ribozymes require a divalent cation, and cleavage results in products with 2', 3'-cyclic phosphate and 5'-OH termini. The *Neurospora* mitochondrial VS RNA *(9)*, a single-stranded circular RNA of 881 nt, shares some features of the self-catalytic RNAs of HDV, group I introns, and some plant viral satellite RNAs. Although VS RNA can be drawn to have a secondary structure like group I introns, it is missing essential basepairing regions, the cleavage site is in a different position, and the termini produced are 2',3'-cyclic phosphate and 5'-OH. Investigations of *trans*-cleavage with the HDV and VS ribozymes have not advanced to those of the hammerhead or hairpin ribozymes.

3. RIBOZYME APPLICATIONS

Ribozymes have been applied as antiviral agents, for the treatment of cancer and genetic disorders, and as tools for pathway elucidation and target validation. Initial uses of ribozymes focused on antiviral, primarily for the treatment of HIV *(31–36)*. Viruses that go through a genomic RNA intermediate in their replication cycle, such as HIV, hepatitis B virus, and hepatitis C virus, are attractive

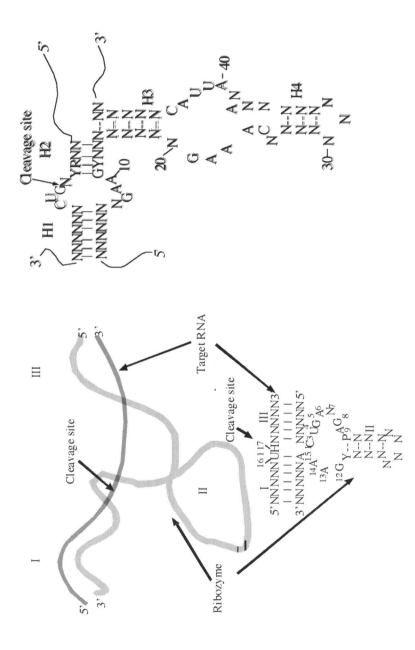

Fig. 1. The hammerhead ribozymes. Secondary structures for the hammerhead ribozyme are depicted: N, any nucleotide; R, purine; and Y, pyrimidine. A diagram of the tertiary structure of the hammerhead ribozyme is depicted above the secondary structure model. The corresponding stems, I, II, and III, in both structures are shown. In the hammerhead ribozyme H, A, C, or U at the cleavage site. In the hairpin ribozymes H1, H2, and the like, refer to the helical regions of the RNA structure.

49

targets because a single species of ribozyme can target both viral genomic RNA and mRNAs. Ribozymes have also been widely used to target cellular genes, including those aberrantly expressed in cancers. One early ribozyme target was the *bcr-abl* fusion transcript created from the Philadelphia chromosome associated with chronic myelogenous leukemia *(37–40)*. This chromosome is characterized by a translocation that results in the expression of a *transforming bcr-abl* fusion protein. In this case, ribozymes have been designed to specifically target the fusion mRNA and not the normal *bcr* or *abl* mRNAs, preventing the function of *bcr–abl* oncogenes. The mutation at codon 12 in c-H-*ras* from GGU to GUU creates a site for hammerhead ribozyme-mediated cleavage. An endogenously expressed ribozyme targeted to this site was effective in preventing focus formation in about 50% of NIH3T3 cells *trans*fected with this activated *ras* gene. In contrast, cells expressing this same ribozyme, but transfected with an activated *ras* in which the codon change was at position 61 instead of 12, were not protected from foci formation by the ribozyme *(41,42)*. Ribozymes targeting overexpressed *HER-2/neu* in breast carcinoma cells effectively reduced the tumorigenicity of these cells in mice*(43,44)*.

In addition to directly targeting oncogenes, ribozymes have also been applied more indirectly as anticancer therapies. For example, ribozymes targeting the multiple drug resistance-1 (MDR1) *(44–46)* or fos mRNAs *(47,48)* in cancer cell lines effectively made the cells more sensitive to chemotherapeutic agents. Alternatively, a ribozyme targeting *bcl-2* triggered apoptosis in oral cancer cells *(49)*. Factors required for metastasis are also attractive targets for ribozymes. Ribozymes targeted against *CAPL/mts (50)* matrix metalloproteinase-9*(51)*, pleiotrophin*(52)*, and VLA-6 integrin *(53,54)* all reduced the metastatic potential of the respective tumor cells. Angiogenesis is also an important target for cancer therapy, and it has been blocked in mice by ribozymes targeting fibroblast growth factor binding protein*(55)* and pleiotrophin*(52)*. Ribozyme-based therapies have also been tested in animals to inhibit other proliferative disorders, such as coronary artery restenosis *(56–58)*. Antitelomerase RNA ribozymes are also being tested for possible applications in cancer gene therapy*(59,60)*. The use of ribozymes as possible therapeutic agents in a variety of cancers has recently been reviewed *(61)*

Heritable and spontaneous genetic disorders represent additional applications for therapeutic ribozymes targeting cellular genes. These include the β-myloid peptide precursor mRNA involved in Alzheimer's disease*(62,63)*, an autosomal-dominant point mutation in the rhodopsin mRNA that gives rise to photoreceptor degeneration and *retinitis pigmentosa (64)*, and *myo*tonic dystrophy *(64a,65–67)*.

4. OPTIMIZING INTRACELLULAR FUNCTION OF RIBOZYMES

In contrast to the rather extensive knowledge of the rules governing ribozyme function in vitro, where free diffusion of ribozyme and target in solution are unrestricted, there are only a limited set of rules for predicting ribozyme efficacy in a complex intracellular environment. The parameters that affect ribozyme function in cells are intracellular stability, expression levels of the ribozyme RNA, intracellular colocalization with the target RNA, stability of the ribozyme transcripts, and interactions of proteins with the ribozymes. The most effective strategies for achieving ribozyme function in vivo involve mechanisms for maximizing the ability the ribozyme to pair with its target RNA. Because the *trans*-cleaving and *trans*-ligation applications of ribozymes involve Watson–Crick basepairing of the ribozyme, or the guide sequence (for RNase P) to the target RNA, this interaction is the rate-limiting step in vivo. Various strategies have been used to identify accessible pairing sites on target RNAs. Not all target sites for these ribozymes are accessible for cleavage: secondary structures, binding of proteins and nucleic acids, and other factors influence intracellular ribozyme efficacy (Fig. 2). Computer-assisted RNA-folding predictions and in vitro cleavage analyses are not necessarily predictive for intracellular or in vivo activity, and the best ribozyme target sites often must be determined empirically in vivo. Strategies utilizing cell extracts with native mRNAs have proven useful for determining accessible ribozyme-binding sites *(68,69)*.

Expression levels and intracellular localization of the ribozyme transcripts are critical for the successful application of the ribozymes in gene therapy. For transcripts, various promoters can be used to obtain either constitutive or regulated expression *(70)*. The transcripts themselves can be engineered to localize within the same cellular or subcellular compartment as the target RNA. For *trans*-cleaving ribozymes to be effective in down-regulating mRNAs, the efficiency of cleavage must be greater than the steady state rates of synthesis and decay of the target (Fig. 3).

For ribozyme down-regulation to be effective, at a given ribozyme concentration the decay mediated by the ribozyme must exceed the steady-state level of target turnover in the absence of ribozyme. This can be best achieved by identifying highly accessible target sites on the target combined with high levels of ribozyme expression in the appropriate cellular compartment. Using these parameters, down-regulation can exceed 90%. A combination of the above elements has been applied to an anti-HIV-1 ribozyme. A ribozyme targeted to a highly accessible and highly conserved site in the HIV genomic and mRNAs was inserted within a small RNA element that directs localization of the transcripts into the nucleolus *(71)*. Because HIV-encoded regulatory proteins Tat and Rev have nucleolar localization signals, and both bind HIV RNA, it was reasoned that these proteins could direct trafficking of HIV RNAs into this organelle. The chimeric ribozyme transcripts were made from a strong Pol III promoter element, producing high levels of the transcript, which localized primarily in the nucleolus. These nucleolar localized ribozymes were positioned to bind and cleave HIV-1 RNAs as they trafficked through the nucleolus, and in fact, they provided

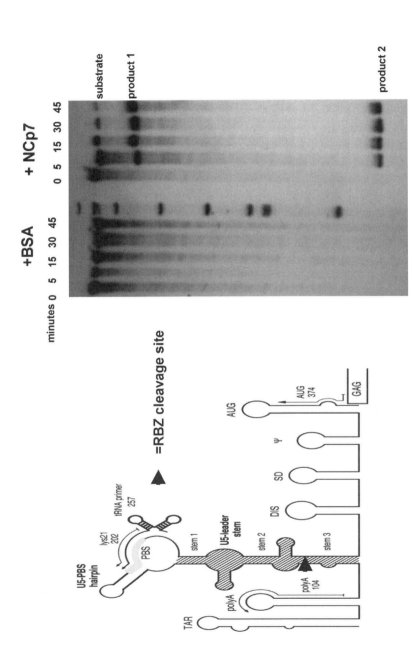

Fig. 2. Protein-mediated facilitation of hammerhead ribozyme cleavage. The HIV-1 encoded peptide NCp7 has an RNP-binding domain and facilitates RNA–RNA interactions. This peptide was incubated in a hammerhead ribozyme cleavage reaction with a long, structured HIV substrate. As a control, the same ribozyme and substrate were incubated with bovine serum albumin at the same concentration as the NCp7. It can be seen that the protein NCp7 greatly facilitates ribozyme cleavage of this long, structured substrate, which ordinarily cannot be cleaved in vitro.

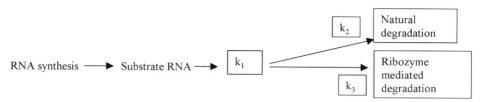

Fig. 3. Kinetics of RNA synthesis and decay impact on ribozyme-mediated turnover.

nearly complete inhibition of HIV replication in cell culture *(71)*. Other strategies for colocalizing ribozymes and substrates to enhance ribozyme function include the use of viral dimerization or packaging domains on ribozyme and target, nuclear versus cytoplasmic localization, and the use of localized mRNA 3' UTRs on ribozyme and target *(70,72–74)*. To achieve maximal ribozyme efficacy, it is important to have some knowledge of the intracellular trafficking of the target RNA. In many instances, the RNAs will not have unique intracellular partitioning, and therefore it becomes necessary to test high levels of ribozyme expression in either the cytoplasm or nucleus to determine which is the best compartment for obtaining optimal ribozyme function.

As the use of ribozymes progresses from cell culture systems into animal models, additional control over ribozyme expression will be required. Ribozyme expression can be restricted to specific organs or cell types through the use of tissue-specific promoters. This has been done successfully in tissue culture using the tyrosinase promoter, which is exclusively expressed in melanocytes *(75)*. In another example, *trans*genic mice that carried a ribozyme gene driven by the insulin promoter were created, and the ribozymes were only expressed in the pancreatic β-cell islets *(76)*. Alternatively, inducible promoters, such as those regulated by tetracycline, have shown utility in both cell culture and in animals, allowing ribozyme expression to be turned on and off at will *(57,77)*.

5. RIBOZYME DELIVERY

Whatever type of ribozyme is chosen, it must be introduced into its target cells. Two general mechanisms exist for introducing catalytic RNA molecules into cells: exogenous delivery of the preformed ribozyme and endogenous expression from a transcriptional unit. Preformed ribozymes can be delivered into cells using liposomes, electroporation, or microinjection. Many exciting developments in the chemical synthesis of RNA and modified forms of RNA have taken place over the past several years. Molecules with long-term stability in serum or intracellular environments have been synthesized *(78–80)*. Several of these backbone-modified ribozymes still maintain the site-specificity and catalytic turnover features of unmodified RNAs, and some have enhanced catalytic properties, making them candidates for ex vivo delivery. Chemically modified ribozymes have been shown to be capable of being delivered without encapsulation and can be taken up by cells *(80)*.

Stable intracellular expression of transcriptionally active ribozymes can be achieved by viral vector-mediated delivery. Currently, retroviral vectors are the most commonly used both in cell culture, primary cells, and transgenic animals *(81)*. Retroviral vectors have the advantage of stable integration into a dividing host cell genome, and the absence of any viral gene expression reduces the chance of an immune response in animals. Additionally, retroviruses can be easily pseudo-typed with a variety of envelope proteins to broaden or restrict host cell tropism, thus adding an additional level of cellular targeting for ribozyme gene delivery. Adenoviral vectors can be produced at high titers and provide very efficient transduction, but they do not integrate into the host genome, and consequently, expression of the transgenes is only *trans*ient in actively dividing cells *(82)*. Other viral delivery systems are actively being pursued, such as the adeno-associated virus, α-viruses, and lentiviruses *(83–89)*. The adeno-associated virus is attractive as a small, nonpathogenic virus that can stably integrate into the host genome. An α-virus system, using recombinant Semliki Forest virus, provides high transduction efficiencies of mammalian cells along with cytoplasmic ribozyme expression *(90)*.

Another vehicle for the ex vivo delivery of ribozyme genes is cationic lipids *(91)*. Because there is a variety of formulations for these lipids, it is usually best to test a panel of lipids for those that provide the highest efficiency of gene transfer with the least toxicity.

6. TRANSGENIC ANIMALS EXPRESSING RIBOZYMES

Therapeutics and target validation studies will certainly be tested in animals. Ribozymes have been used in transgenic mice to create disease models such as diabetes by selectively down-regulating the hexokinase mRNA in pancreatic islets *(76)*. In this case, the ribozyme expression was under the control of the insulin promoter and was therefore only expressed in the pancreatic β-cells. Retroviral delivery of ribozymes targeted against neuregulin-1 in a chick blastoderm resulted in the same embryonic lethal phenotype as a gene knockout *(92)*. Localized retroviral delivery of the same ribozyme later in development allowed dissection of the neuregulin biochemical pathway *(93)*. The use of a heat inducible ribozyme against *Fushi tarzu* in *Drosophila* allowed the developmentally timed disruption of this gene function in *Drosophila* embryos *(94)*.

7. RIBOZYME-MEDIATED RNA REPAIR

A novel therapeutic application of ribozymes exploits the *trans*-splicing activity of the *Tetrahymena* ribozyme. This ribozyme has been used to repair

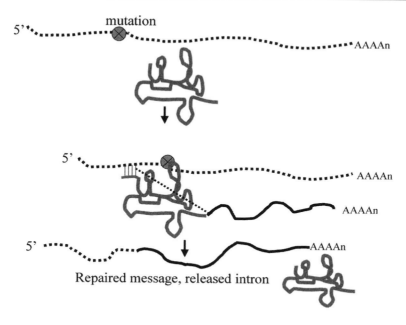

Fig. 4. The group I intron catalyzes a *trans*-splicing reaction. A modified version of the group I intron can be used to *trans*-splice a piece of message to a defective transcript. The target binds to the modified internal guide sequence of the intron. The 3' exon is trans-spliced to the target message, generating a new transcript and a released intron.

defective mRNAs by *trans*-splicing onto these RNAs a functional sequence (*16, 95*) (Fig. 4). These ribozymes are designed to bind and cleave the target RNAs 5' of the undesired mutation. Because the ribozyme in this case is an intron, it is engineered to carry with it the correct RNA sequence as the 3' exon. Following cleavage of the mutant target RNA, the ribozyme catalyzes ligation of the wild-type sequence onto the cleaved transcript. This was first successfully demonstrated with the correction of a mutant *lacZ* transcript (*16*) in bacteria and subsequently correction of a sickle cell message in erythroid cells (*96*).

8. RIBOZYME EVOLUTION

The discovery of the ribozyme sparked new debate on the "RNA world" hypothesis, wherein all biological processes are carried out by RNA-based enzymes. Since then, RNA evolution has been forced in vitro to come up with RNA enzymes capable of carrying out a wide variety of biochemical reactions, as far-reaching as carbon–carbon bond and peptide bond formation. In vitro RNA evolution has been used to create RNA-cleaving ribozymes with smaller catalytic domains, DNA-cleaving ribozymes, and new catalytic motifs (*97*).

Part II / Basic Methodology

Table I. Partial List of Successful Ribozyme-Mediated Target mRNA Downregulation

Target	Effect	Reference
HIV-1	Block viral replication in vitro	33,103
CCR5	Block HIV-1 cell entry in vitro	103,104
Chronic myelogenous leukemia bcr/abl mRNA	Block cell proliferation in vitro	37,39,40,105
Ras	Block tumor foci formation in vitro and in vivo	106,107
Her2/neu	Block tumorigenicity in vivo	55,108
MDR1 Cfos	Make cells more sensitive to chemotherapeutic agents in vitro	44–46,48,49,55,108–110
Bcl2	Trigger apoptosis in vitro	50–54
CAPL/mts MMP9 Pleiotrophin VLA-6 integrin FGFBP	Reduce or eliminate metastatic potential of cells in vivo	43,52,54,111–116
VegF Receptor	Block angiogenesis in vitro and in vivo	43,111,114,116
PNA1 c-Myb Lipoxygenase β-amyloid peptide	Block restenosis in vivo	58,117,118
mRNA	Block amyloid plaque formation in vitro	62,63
Rhodopsin	Block photoreceptor degeneration in vivo	64,119–121
Ftz	Block pattern formation in vivo	94
Hexokinase	Generate type II diabetes model in vivo	76

Even RNA-cleaving DNAzymes have been generated through in vitro evolution (98). These "evolved" enzymes exemplify the power of in vitro evolution and will no doubt find many applications.

It is reasonable to conclude that achieving effective ribozyme–substrate interactions and ribozyme function in an intracellular environment is not a straightforward task, and that new strategies for expression and localization of ribozymes in the intracellular milieu will be required to permit the general utility of ribozymes as therapeutic agents.

9. OTHER CONSIDERATIONS

Although basepairing specificity confers target selectivity, minimizing the potential for general toxicity, the question of toxicity must be rigorously tested because mispairing by a ribozyme to a nontargeted substrate could elicit undesired antisense inhibitory effects. Because every ribozyme sequence has different potential basepairing interactions, an accumulation of data from many different ribozyme experiments will be required to rigorously assess this potential problem. Some of the potential sources of toxicity are nonspecific interactions of ribozymes with cellular proteins, the generation of high intracellular concentrations of the cleavage products, and the inhibitory effects on cellular metabolism of various chemically generated backbone modifications used to stabilize presynthesized ribozymes.

A different problem is loss of ribozyme activity due to basepairing mismatches or mutations at the site of cleavage. This is an especially significant problem in designing ribozymes against genetically variable targets such as HIV. By choosing targets in highly conserved sequences and simultaneously using multiple ribozymes to a number of targets, loss of ribozyme activity can be minimized. Such strategies are already being tested by a number of laboratories.

One of the potential advantages of ribozymes versus antisense RNAs is their catalytic activity, which could theoretically lead to inactivation of multiple targeted substrates. It has yet to be demonstrated that this type of catalytic activity can occur intracellularly. Protein facilitation of hammerhead ribozyme-mediated cleavage *(99–101)* suggests that intracellular ribozyme mediated substrate turnover may be possible. Experiments designed to exploit the protein facilitation of ribozyme turnover intracellularly are currently underway in several laboratories. The inclusion of RNA-binding proteins in in vitro evolution strategies to enrich for ribozyme–protein combinations with enhanced catalytical activities should also be exploited. Finally, the design and chemical synthesis of ribozymes capable of high catalytic turnover as a consequence of specific base and backbone modifications is a distinct possibility.

10. FUTURE PROSPECTS

The notion that ribozymes could be used as therapeutic agents has only been around for a few years, yet there is a great deal of interest in deploying clinically useful ribozymes in the very near future. At this time it is premature to conclude that ribozymes will have a place in the repertoire of therapeutic agents available to modern medicine. We must learn a great deal more about the movement of RNA inside the cells as well as the cellular factors that can impede or enhance ribozyme utilization. These are not simple problems, and they are not confined to those studying the application of ribozymes. As techniques in cell biology become more refined, answers to some of these problems will be forthcoming.

The transformation of ribozyme sequences from naturally occurring, *cis*-cleaving (and ligating) molecules to target-specific, *trans*-cleaving (and ligating) reagents has stimulated a great deal of interest in their potential applications. Ribozymes targeting viral genes are now in clinical evaluation; ribozymes targeting cellular genes are moving into transgenic animals; and the use of ribozymes is expanding into RNA evolution, mRNA repair, and gene discovery.

For ribozymes to become realistic therapeutic agents, several obstacles first need to be overcome. These obstacles are the efficient delivery to a high percentage of the cell population, efficient expression of the ribozyme from a vector or intracellular ribozyme concentration, colocalization of the ribozyme with the target, specificity of ribozyme for the desired mRNA, and an enhancement of ribozyme-mediated substrate turnover. As our knowledge of RNA structure, secondary and tertiary, increases, we will be able to target RNAs more rationally, which may help with the problems of specificity. At the same time, the understanding of the physical localization of RNA in cells and its tracking as it moves from the nucleus to cytoplasm will also help in ensuring colocalization of the ribozyme and target. Modifications of the ribozymes, for example, the 2' ribose with various agents such as methyl, allyl, fluoro, and amino groups, increase the stability to nucleases quite dramatically. Similarly, chimeric DNA–RNA ribozymes increase the stability. The efficiency of delivery to cells with viral vectors or liposomes is also continually improving. These molecules must retain their catalytic potential, reach an accessible site on the substrate, and effectively impact the steady-state levels of target molecules to be useful as either surrogate genetic tools or as therapeutic agents. Great progress has been made in all of these areas and should allow extensive use of the highly specific reagents for down-regulating expression of target RNAs.

ACKNOWLEDGMENTS

The author was supported by NIH grants AI 29329 and AI 42552.

REFERENCES

1. Kruger K, Grabowski PJ, Zaug AJ, Sands J, Gottschling DE, Cech TR. Self-splicing RNA: autoexcision and autocyclization of the ribosomal RNA intervening sequence of tetrahymena. Cell 1982; 31:147.
2. Bevilacqua PC, Turner DH. Comparison of binding of mixed ribose-deoxyribose analogues of CUCU to a ribozyme and to GGAGAA by equilibrium dialysis: evidence for ribozyme specific interactions with 2' OH groups. Biochemistry 1991; 30:10632.
3. Guerrier-Takada C, Gardiner K, Marsh T, Pace N, Altman S. The RNA moiety of ribonuclease P is the catalytic subunit of the enzyme. Cell 1983; 35:849–857.
4. Costa M, Michel F. Frequent use of the same tertiary motif by self-folding RNAs. Embo J 1995; 14:1276.

5. Hutchins CJ, Rathjen PD, Forster AC, Symons RH. Self-cleavage of plus and minus RNA transcripts of avocado sunblotch viroid. Nucleic Acids Res 1986; 14:3627.

6. Buzayan, JM McNinch JS, Schneider IR, Bruening G. A nucleotide sequence rearrangement distinguishes two isolates of satellite tobacco ringspot virus RNA. Virology 1987; 160:95.

7. Buzayan JM, Hampel A, Bruening G. Nucleotide sequence and newly formed phosphodiester bond of spontaneously ligated satellite tobacco ringspot virus RNA. Nucleic Acids Res 1986; 14:9729.

8. Kumar PK, Suh YA, Miyashiro H, et al. Random mutations to evaluate the role of bases at two important single- stranded regions of genomic HDV ribozyme. Nucleic Acids Res 1992; 20:3919.

9. Saville BJ, Collins RA. A site-specific self-cleavage reaction performed by a novel RNA in Neurospora mitochondria. Cell 1990; 61:685.

10. Cech TR. Structural biology. The ribosome is a ribozyme. Science 2000; 289:878.

11. Moore PB, Steitz TA. After the ribosome structures: How does peptidyl transferase work? RNA 2003; 9:155.

12. Nissen P, Hansen J, Ban N, Moore PB, Steitz TA. The structural basis of ribosome activity in peptide bond synthesis. Science 2000; 289:920.

13. Setlik RF, Shibata M, Sarma RH, et al. Modeling of a possible conformational change associated with the catalytic mechanism in the hammerhead ribozyme. J Biomol Struct Dyn 1995; 13:515.

14. Wilson DS, Szostak JW. In vitro selection of functional nucleic acids. Annu Rev Biochem 1999; 68:611.

15. Bartel DP, Doudna JA, Usman N, Szostak JW. Template-directed primer extension catalyzed by the tetrahymena ribozyme. Mol Cell Biol 1991; 11:3390.

16. Sullenger BA, Cech TR. Ribozyme-mediated repair of defective mRNA by targeted, trans-splicing. Nature 1994; 371:619.

17. Watanabe T, Sullenger BA. Induction of wild-type p53 activity in human cancer cells by ribozymes that repair mutant p53 transcripts. Proc Natl Acad Sci USA 2000; 97:8490.

18. Guo H, Karberg M, Long M, Jones JP, III, Sullenger B, Lambowitz AM. Group II introns designed to insert into therapeutically relevant DNA target sites in human cells. Science 2000; 289:452.

19. Kurz JC, Fierke CA. Ribonuclease P: a ribonucleoprotein enzyme. Curr Opin Chem Biol 2000; 4:553.

20. Forster AC, Altman S. External guide sequences for an RNA enzyme. Science 1990; 249:783.

21. Ikawa Y, Shiraishi H, Inoue T. Trans-activation of the tetrahymena ribozyme by its P2-2.1 domains. J Biochem (Tokyo) 1998; 123:528.

22. Duhamel J, Liu DM, Evilia C, Fleysh N, Dinter-Gottlieb G, Lu P. Secondary structure content of the HDV ribozyme in 95% formamide. Nucleic Acids Res 1996; 24:3911.

23. Trang P, Kilani A, Lee J, et al. RNase P ribozymes for the studies and treatment of human cytomegalovirus infections. J Clin Virol 2002; 25 Suppl 2:S63.

24. Trang P, Lee J, Kilani AF, Kim J, Liu F. Effective inhibition of herpes simplex virus 1 gene expression and growth by engineered RNase P ribozyme. Nucleic Acids Res 2001; 29:5071.

25. Trang P, Hsu A, Zhou T, et al. Engineered RNase P ribozymes inhibit gene expression and growth of cytomegalovirus by increasing rate of cleavage and substrate binding. J Mol Biol 2002; 315:573.

26. Trang P, Lee M, Nepomuceno E, Kim J, Zhu H, Liu F. Effective inhibition of human cytomegalovirus gene expression and replication by a ribozyme derived from the catalytic RNA subunit of RNase P from Escherichia coli. Proc Natl Acad Sci USA 2000; 97:5812.

27. Forster AC, Jeffries AC, Sheldon CC, Symons RH. Structural and ionic requirements for self-cleavage of virusoid RNAs and trans self-cleavage of viroid RNA. Cold Spring Harb Symp Quant Biol 1987; 52:249.
28. Haseloff J, Gerlach WL. Simple RNA enzymes with new and highly specific endoribonuclease activities. 1988 [classical article]. Biotechnology 1992; 24:264.
29. Hampel A, Tritz R, Hicks M, Cruz P. Nucleic Acids Research 1990; 18:299–304.
30. Perrotta AT, Been MD. Assessment of disparate structural features in three models of the hepatitis delta virus ribozyme. Nucleic Acids Res 1993; 21:3959.
31. Rossi JJ. Ribozyme therapy for HIV infection. Adv Drug Deliv Rev 2000; 44:71.
32. Rossi JJ. The application of ribozymes to HIV infection. Curr Opin Mol Ther 1999; 1:316.
33. Rossi JJ, Cantin EM, Zaia JA, et al. Ribozymes as therapies for AIDS. Ann N Y Acad Sci 1990; 616:184.
34. Sarver N, Cantin EM, Chang PS, et al. Ribozymes as potential anti-HIV-1 therapeutic agents. Science 1990; 247:1222.
35. Rossi JJ, Sarver N. RNA enzymes (ribozymes) as antiviral therapeutic agents. Trends Biotechnol 1990; 8:179.
36. Lee NS, Bertrand E, Rossi J. mRNA localization signals can enhance the intracellular effectiveness of hammerhead ribozymes. RNA 1999; 5:1200.
37. Snyder DS, Wu Y, McMahon R, Yu L, Rossi JJ, Forman SJ. Ribozyme-mediated inhibition of a Philadelphia chromosome-positive acute lymphoblastic leukemia cell line expressing the p190 bcr-abl oncogene. Biol Blood Marrow Transplant 1997; 3:179.
38. Kuwabara T, Warashina M, Orita M, Koseki S, Ohkawa J, Taira K. Formation of a catalytically active dimer by tRNA(Val)-driven short ribozymes. Nat Biotechnol 1998; 16:961.
39. Lange W. Cleavage of BCR/ABL mRNA by synthetic ribozymes—effects on the proliferation rate of K562 cells. Klin Padiatr 1995; 207:222.
40. Snyder DS, Wu Y, Wang JL, et al. Ribozyme-mediated inhibition of bcr-abl gene expression in a Philadelphia chromosome-positive cell line. Blood 1993; 82:600.
41. Hertel KJ, Pardi A, Uhlenbeck OC, et al. Numbering system for the hammerhead. Nucleic Acids Res 1992; 20:3252.
42. Kijima H, Tsuchida T, Kondo H, et al. Hammerhead ribozymes against gamma-glutamylcysteine synthetase mRNA down-regulate intracellular glutathione concentration of mouse islet cells. Biochem Biophys Res Commun 1998; 247:697.
43. Czubayko F, Liaudet-Coopman ED, Aigner A, Tuveson AT, Berchem GJ, Wellstein A. A secreted FGF-binding protein can serve as the angiogenic switch in human cancer [see comments]. Nat Med 1997; 3:1137.
44. Kobayashi H, Dorai T, Holland JF, Ohnuma T. Reversal of drug sensitivity in multidrug-resistant tumor cells by an MDR1 (PGY1) ribozyme. Cancer Res 1994; 54:1271.
45. Scanlon KJ, Ishida H, Kashani-Sabet M. Ribozyme-mediated reversal of the multidrug-resistant phenotype. Proc Natl Acad Sci USA 1994; 91:11123.
46. Wang FS, Kobayashi H, Liang KW, Holland JF, Ohnuma T. Retrovirus-mediated transfer of anti-MDR1 ribozymes fully restores chemosensitivity of P-glycoprotein-expressing human lymphoma cells. Hum Gene Ther 1999; 10:1185.
47. Funato T, Shitara T, Tone T, Jiao L, Kashani-Sabet M, Scanlon KJ. Suppression of H-ras-mediated transformation in NIH3T3 cells by a *ras* ribozyme. Biochem Pharmacol 1994; 48:1471.

48. Funato T. [Circumventing multidrug resistance in human cancer by anti-ribozyme]. Nippon Rinsho 1997; 55:1116.
49. Gibson SA, Pellenz C, Hutchison RE, Davey FR, Shillitoe EJ. Induction of apoptosis in oral cancer cells by an anti-bcl-2 ribozyme delivered by an adenovirus vector. Clin Cancer Res 2000; 6:213.
50. Maelandsmo GM, Hovig E, Skrede M, et al. Reversal of the in vivo metastatic phenotype of human tumor cells by an anti-CAPL (mts1) ribozyme. Cancer Res 1996; 56:5490.
51. Sehgal G, Hua J, Bernhard EJ, Sehgal I, Thompson TC, Muschel RJ. Requirement for matrix metalloproteinase-9 (gelatinase B) expression in metastasis by murine prostate carcinoma. Am J Pathol 1998; 152:591.
52. Czubayko F, Riegel AT, Wellstein A. Ribozyme-targeting elucidates a direct role of pleiotrophin in tumor growth. J Biol Chem 1994; 269:21358.
53. Yamamoto H, Irie A, Fukushima Y, et al. Abrogation of lung metastasis of human fibrosarcoma cells by ribozyme-mediated suppression of integrin alpha6 subunit expression. Int J Cancer 1996; 65:519.
54. Feng B, Rollo EE, Denhardt DT. Osteopontin (OPN) may facilitate metastasis by protecting cells from macrophage NO-mediated cytotoxicity: evidence from cell lines down- regulated for OPN expression by a targeted ribozyme. Clin Exp Metastasis 1995; 13:453.
55. Czubayko F, Downing SG, Hsieh SS, et al. Adenovirus-mediated transduction of ribozymes abrogates HER-2/neu and pleiotrophin expression and inhibits tumor cell proliferation. Gene Ther 1997; 4:943.
56. Frimerman A, Welch PJ, Jin X, et al. Chimeric DNA-RNA hammerhead ribozyme to proliferating cell nuclear antigen reduces stent-induced stenosis in a porcine coronary model. Circulation 1999; 99:697.
57. Gu JL, Pei H, Thomas L, et al. Ribozyme-mediated inhibition of rat leukocyte-type 12-lipoxygenase prevents intimal hyperplasia in balloon-injured rat carotid arteries. Circulation 2001; 103:1446.
58. Jarvis TC, Alby LJ, Beaudry AA, et al. Inhibition of vascular smooth muscle cell proliferation by ribozymes that cleave c-myb mRNA. RNA 1996; 2:419.
59. Saretzki G, Ludwig A, von Zglinicki T, Runnebaum IB. Ribozyme-mediated telomerase inhibition induces immediate cell loss but not telomere shortening in ovarian cancer cells. Cancer Gene Ther 2001; 8:827.
60. Yokoyama Y, Wan X, Shinohara A, Takahashi Y, Tamaya T. Hammerhead ribozymes to modulate telomerase activity of endometrial carcinoma cells. Hum Cell 2001; 14:223.
61. Kashani-Sabet M. Ribozyme therapeutics. J Investig Dermatol Symp Proc 2002; 7:76.
62. Dolzhanskaya N, Conti J, Merz G, Denman RB. In vivo ribozyme targeting of betaAPP+ mRNAs. Mol Cell Biol Res Commun 2000; 4:239.
63. Currie JR, Chen-Hwang MC, Denman R, et al. Reduction of histone cytotoxicity by the Alzheimer beta-amyloid peptide precursor. Biochim Biophys Acta 1997; 1355:248.
64. LaVail MM, Yasumura D, Matthes MT, et al. Ribozyme rescue of photoreceptor cells in P23H transgenic rats: long-term survival and late-stage therapy. Proc Natl Acad Sci USA 2000; 97:11488.
64a. Langlois MA, Lee NS, Rossi JJ, Paymirat J. Hammerhead ribozyme mediated destruction of nuclear foci in myotonic dystrophy myoblasts. Mol Ther 2003; 7:670.
65. Phylactou LA, Darrah C, Wood MJ. Ribozyme-mediated trans-splicing of a trinucleotide repeat. Nat Genet 1998; 18:378.
66. Bell MA, Johnson AK, Testa SM. Ribozyme-catalyzed excision of targeted sequences from within RNAs. Biochemistry 2002; 41:15327.

67. Rossi JJ. Ribozymes to the rescue: repairing genetically defective mRNAs. Trends Genet 1998; 14:295.
68. Castanotto D, Scherr M, Rossi JJ. Intracellular expression and function of antisense catalytic RNAs. Methods Enzymol 2000; 313:401.
69. Scherr M, Rossi JJ. Rapid determination and quantitation of the accessibility to native RNAs by antisense oligodeoxynucleotides in murine cell extracts. Nucleic Acids Res 1998; 26:5079.
70. Bertrand E, Castanotto D, Zhou C, et al. The expression cassette determines the functional activity of ribozymes in mammalian cells by controlling their intracellular localization. RNA 1997; 3:75.
71. Michienzi A, Cagnon L, Bahner I, Rossi JJ. Ribozyme-mediated inhibition of HIV 1 suggests nucleolar trafficking of HIV-1 RNA. Proc Natl Acad Sci USA 2000; 97:8955.
72. Sullenger BA, Cech TR. Tethering ribozymes to a retroviral packaging signal for destruction of viral RNA. Science 1993; 262:1566.
73. Sullenger BA. Colocalizing ribozymes with substrate RNAs to increase their efficacy as gene inhibitors. Appl Biochem Biotechnol 1995; 54:57.
74. Good PD, Krikos AJ, Li SX, et al. Expression of small, therapeutic RNAs in human cell nuclei. Gene Ther 1997; 4:45.
75. Ohta Y, Kijima H, Kashani-Sabet M, Scanlon KJ. Suppression of the malignant phenotype of melanoma cells by anti-oncogene ribozymes. J Invest Dermatol 1996; 106:275.
76. Efrat S, Leiser M, Wu YJ, et al. Ribozyme-mediated attenuation of pancreatic beta-cell glucokinase expression in transgenic mice results in impaired glucose-induced insulin secretion. Proc Natl Acad Sci USA 1994; 91:2051.
77. Benedict CM, Pan W, Loy SE, Clawson GA. Triple ribozyme-mediated down-regulation of the retinoblastoma gene. Carcinogenesis 1998; 19:1223.
78. Heidenreich O, Benseler F, Fahrenholz A, Eckstein F. High activity and stability of hammerhead ribozymes containing 2'- modified pyrimidine nucleosides and phosphorothioates. J Biol Chem 1994; 269:2131.
79. Burgin AB, Jr, Gonzalez C, Matulic-Adamic J, et al. Chemically modified hammerhead ribozymes with improved catalytic rates. Biochemistry 1996; 35:14090.
80. Flory CM, Pavco PA, Jarvis TC, et al. Nuclease-resistant ribozymes decrease stromelysin mRNA levels in rabbit synovium following exogenous delivery to the knee joint. Proc Natl Acad Sci USA 1996; 93:754.
81. Morgan RA, Anderson WF. Human gene therapy. Annu Rev Biochem 1993; 62:191.
82. Perlman H, Sata M, Krasinski K, Dorai T, Buttyan R, Walsh K. Adenovirus-encoded hammerhead ribozyme to Bcl-2 inhibits neointimal hyperplasia and induces vascular smooth muscle cell apoptosis. Cardiovasc Res 2000; 45:570.
83. Giordano V, Jin DY, Rekosh D, Jeang KT. Intravirion targeting of a functional anti-human immunodeficiency virus ribozyme directed to pol. Virology 2000; 267:174.
84. Horster A, Teichmann B, Hormes R, Grimm D, Kleinschmidt J, Sczakiel G. Recombinant AAV-2 harboring gfp-antisense/ribozyme fusion sequences monitor transduction, gene expression, and show anti-HIV-1 efficacy. Gene Ther 1999; 6:1231.
85. Kunke D, Grimm D, Denger S, et al. Preclinical study on gene therapy of cervical carcinoma using adeno-associated virus vectors. Cancer Gene Ther 2000; 7:766.
86. L'Huillier PJ, Davis SR, Bellamy AR. Cytoplasmic delivery of ribozymes leads to efficient reduction in alpha-lactalbumin mRNA levels in C127I mouse cells. Embo J 1992; 11:4411.
87. Lipkowitz MS, Hanss B, Tulchin N, et al. Transduction of renal cells in vitro and in vivo by adeno-associated virus gene therapy vectors. J Am Soc Nephrol 1999; 10:1908.
88. Sczakiel G, Pawlita M. Inhibition of human immunodeficiency virus type 1 replication in human T-cells stably expressing antisense RNA. J Virol 1991; 65:468.
89. Welch PJ, Yei S, Barber JR. Ribozyme gene therapy for hepatitis C virus infection. Clin Diagn Virol 1998; 10:163.

90. Smith SM, Maldarelli F, Jeang KT. Efficient expression by an alphavirus replicon of a functional ribozyme targeted to human immunodeficiency virus type 1. J Virol 1997; 71:9713.

91. Castanotto D, Chow WA, Li H, Rossi JJ. Unusual interactions between cleavage products of a cis-cleaving hammerhead ribozyme. Antisense Nucleic Acid Drug Dev 1998; 8:499.

92. Tang CK, Goldstein DJ, Payne J, et al. ErbB-4 ribozymes abolish neuregulin-induced mitogenesis. Cancer Res 1998; 58:3415.

93. Zhao JJ, Lemke G. Selective disruption of neuregulin-1 function in vertebrate embryos using ribozyme-tRNA transgenes. Development 1998; 125:1899.

94. Zhao JJ, Pick L. Generating loss-of-function phenotypes of the fushi tarazu gene with a targeted ribozyme in Drosophila. Nature 1993; 365:448.

95. Watanabe T, Sullenger BA. RNA repair: a novel approach to gene therapy. Adv Drug Deliv Rev 2000; 44:109.

96. Chaulk SG, MacMillan AM. Caged RNA: photo-control of a ribozyme reaction. Nucleic Acids Res 1998; 26:3173.

97. Hager AJ, Szostak JW. Isolation of novel ribozymes that ligate AMP-activated RNA substrates. Chem Biol 1997; 4:607.

98. Santoro SW, Joyce GF. Mechanism and utility of an RNA-cleaving DNA enzyme. Biochemistry 1998; 37:13330.

99. Coetzee T, Herschlag D, Belfort M. Escherichia coli proteins, including ribosomal protein S12, facilitate in vitro splicing of phage T4 introns by acting as RNA chaperones. Genes Dev 1994; 8:1575.

100. Bertrand E, Pictet R, Grange T. Can hammerhead ribozymes be efficient tools to inactivate gene function? [published erratum appears in Nucleic Acids Res 1994; 22(7):1326]. Nucleic Acids Res 1994; 22:293.

101. Sioud M, Jespersen L. Enhancement of hammerhead ribozyme catalysis by glyceraldehyde-3-phosphate dehydrogenase. J Mol Biol 1996; 257:775.

102. Yu M, Ojwang J, Yamada O, et al. A hairpin ribozyme inhibits expression of diverse strains of human immunodeficiency virus type 1 [published erratum appears in Proc Natl Acad Sci USA 1993; 90(17):8303]. Proc Natl Acad Sci USA 1993; 90:6340.

103. Bai J, Gorantla S, Banda N, Cagnon L, Rossi J, Akkina R. Characterization of anti-CCR5 ribozyme-transduced CD34+ hematopoietic progenitor cells in vitro and in a SCID-hu mouse model in vivo. Mol Ther 2000; 1:244.

104. Bai J, Rossi J, Akkina R. Multivalent anti-CCR ribozymes for stem cell-based HIV type 1 gene therapy. AIDS Res Hum Retroviruses 2001; 17:385.

105. Kuwabara T, Warashina M, Tanabe T, Tani K, Asano S, Taira K. A novel allosterically transactivated ribozyme, the maxizyme, with exceptional specificity in vitro and in vivo. Mol Cell 1998; 2:617.

106. Koizumi M, Ohtsuka E. Design of RNAs that inhibit the activated c-Ha-ras gene in mammalian cells. Ann N Y Acad Sci 1992; 660:276.

107. Tsuchida T, Kijima H, Hori S, et al. Adenovirus-mediated anti-K-ras ribozyme induces apoptosis and growth suppression of human pancreatic carcinoma. Cancer Gene Ther 2000; 7:373.

108. Lui VW, He Y, Huang L. Specific down-regulation of HER-2/neu mediated by a chimeric U6 hammerhead ribozyme results in growth inhibition of human ovarian carcinoma. Mol Ther 2001; 3:169.

109. Scanlon KJ, Jiao L, Funato T, et al. Ribozyme-mediated cleavage of c-fos mRNA reduces gene expression of DNA synthesis enzymes and metallothionein. Proc Natl Acad Sci USA 1991; 88:10591.

110. Funato T. [Reversal of drug resistance in human cancer cells by anti-oncogenes]. Gan To Kagaku Ryoho 1997; 24:395.
111. Czubayko F, Schulte AM, Berchem GJ, Wellstein A. Melanoma angiogenesis and metastasis modulated by ribozyme targeting of the secreted growth factor pleiotrophin. Proc Natl Acad Sci USA 1996; 93:14753.
112. Gibson I. Antisense approaches to the gene therapy of cancer—"Recnac." Cancer Metastasis Rev 1996; 15:287.
113. Wellstein A, Czubayko F. Inhibition of fibroblast growth factors. Breast Cancer Res Treat 1996; 38:109.
114. Pavco PA, Bouhana KS, Gallegos AM, et al. Antitumor and antimetastatic activity of ribozymes targeting the messenger RNA of vascular endothelial growth factor receptors. Clin Cancer Res 2000; 6:2094.
115. Ho JJ, Kim YS. Biliopancreatic malignancy: future prospects for progress. Ann Oncol 1999; 10(Suppl 4):300.
116. Czubayko F, Liaudet-Coopman ED, Aigner A, Tuveson AT, Berchem GJ, Wellstein A. A secreted FGF-binding protein can serve as the angiogenic switch in human cancer. Nat Med 1997; 3:1137.
117. Jarvis TC, Wincott FE, Alby LJ, et al. Optimizing the cell efficacy of synthetic ribozymes. Site selection and chemical modifications of ribozymes targeting the proto-oncogene c-myb. J Biol Chem 1996; 271:29107.
118. Putnam DA. Antisense strategies and therapeutic applications [published erratum appears in Am J Health Syst Pharm 1996; 53(3):325]. Am J Health Syst Pharm 1996; 53:151.
119. Fritz JJ, White DA, Lewin AS, Hauswirth WW. Designing and characterizing hammer-head ribozymes for use in AAV vector-mediated retinal gene therapies. Methods Enzymol 2002; 346:358.
120. Hauswirth WW, Lewin AS. Ribozyme uses in retinal gene therapy. Prog Retin Eye Res 2000; 19:689.
121. Hauswirth WW, LaVail MM, Flannery JG, Lewin AS. Ribozyme gene therapy for autosomal dominant retinal disease. Clin Chem Lab Med 2000; 38:147.

5 Use of Catalytic DNA in Target Validation and Therapeutics

Lun-Quan Sun, *PhD*

CONTENTS

INTRODUCTION
IN VITRO CATALYTIC ACTIVITY
TARGET SITE SELECTION
CONCLUSION
REFERENCES

1. INTRODUCTION

RNA is a relatively amenable target for nucleic-acid-based gene suppression, because it is transcribed in a single-stranded form from its parent double-helical DNA. The unpaired bases of this polynucleotide are therefore in theory available for hybridization by other complementary single-stranded nucleic acids such as antisense reagents. Where these hybridization events impair the ability of the RNA to function, for example, in translation, they can bring about suppression of the genes' expression. Probably the most common mechanism for oligonucleotide-based suppression is heteroduplex-mediated induction of RNase H, which digests the RNA component of the hybrid, leaving the DNA to bind to other target molecules *(1)*. In an alternative strategy, catalytic RNA such as the hammerhead ribozyme, which has its own built-in RNA cleavage activity, can be used to bind and destroy target RNA *(2)*. These have the advantage of being independent of RNase H; however, they lack the natural chemical and biological stability possessed by the antisense DNA oligonucleotide (ON). Although it is possible to manufacture biologically active RNA, its relative fragility in this environment makes it difficult to administer in a direct delivery mode. For this and other reasons, most ribozyme applications rely on transgenic production of RNA in vivo within the context of a gene therapy.

From: *Cancer Drug Discovery and Development:*
Nucleic Acid Therapeutics in Cancer
Edited by: A. M. Gewirtz © Humana Press Inc., Totowa, NJ

65

An ideal oligonucleotide-based gene inactivation agent targeting RNA would possibly combine the self-sufficient RNA digestion capability of ribozymes such as the hammerhead and the hairpin, with the biological resilience of the antisense ON. In nature, the relative stability of double-helical DNA and its ability to replicate with high fidelity make it well suited for storage and transmission of genetic information. DNA secondary and tertiary structure in these systems, however, is severely restricted by its double-stranded nature and provides very little opportunity for the exploration of conformations, which might facilitate useful reaction rate enhancement. Although DNA molecules with RNA cleavage activity have not been observed in nature, some have been derived as a result of an artificial evolutionary system known as in vitro selection *(3–5)*. In an in vitro selection system, DNA liberated from its complementary strand is free to explore a full range of structural possibilities, some of which have been found to be capable of catalytic activity, including site-specific RNA cleavage and ligation *(6,7)*. Among these catalytic DNA molecules, 10–23 DNAzyme has attracted a great attention for its catalytic efficiency and versatile properties for biological applications.

The 10–23 RNA-cleaving DNAzyme is a catalytic nucleic acid composed entirely of DNA (Fig. 1) *(5)*. It was derived from a combinatorial library of sequences by in vitro selection. The tremendous activity and sequence specificity against its target RNA's undersimulated physiological condition *(8,9)* has generated the expectation that it may function in cells as a gene suppression agent. In this chapter we will describe some kinetic features and design rules for this molecule. We will also discuss the potential use of the DNAzyme in gene regulation and detection. Finally, we will highlight some aspects in use of the DNAzyme for target validation.

2. IN VITRO CATALYTIC ACTIVITY

The ability of the 10–23 DNAzyme to cleave purine–pyrimidine junctions meant that the AUG start codon of any gene could be used as a target. Early kinetic analysis of the 10–23 DNAzyme focused on synthetic substrate sequences derived from the start codons of various HIV genes *(5)*. A key point that emerged from this analysis was that the kinetic efficiency of DNAzyme catalyzed cleavage varied substantially from one substrate sequence to the next. This sequence-dependent variability seemed to be closely associated with the thermodynamic stability of the enzyme-substrate heteroduplex as predicted by the hybridization-free energy *(10)*. In this relationship, DNA enzymes with the greatest heteroduplex stability, indicated by a low free energy of hybridization (calculated using the nearest neighbor method), were often found to have the greatest kinetic activity. The sensitivity to heteroduplex stability in most instances can be counterbalanced to some extent by increasing the arm length until the hybridization

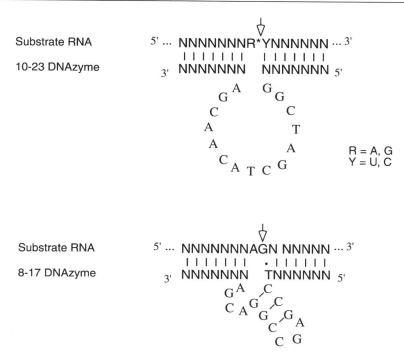

Fig. 1. A schematic representation of the 10–23 and 8–17 general-purpose RNA cleaving deoxyribozymes. Panels A and B contain illustrations of the 10–23 and 8–17 deoxyribozymes, respectively. Watson–Crick interactions for each deoxyribozyme–substrate complex are represented by generic ribonucleotides (N) in the target (top) and the corresponding deoxyribonucleotides (N) in the arms of the deoxyribozyme (bottom) of each. The defined sequences in the loop joining the arms and spanning a single unpaired purine at the RNA target site of each model represent the conserved catalytic motif.

free energy decreases to a threshold level. At this point, the heteroduplex stability is optimal for catalysis, and the enzyme activity can approach its maximum efficiency. Factors other than length, which tend to increase the heteroduplex stability, include the general GC content and specific pyrimidine content of the DNA (10–12). The influence of heteroduplex stability on the kinetic efficiency of the DNAzyme is probably derived from its effect on the K_M of the reaction. The inverse relationship between K_M and enzyme-substrate complex stability can be observed by increasing the substrate binding domain length such that the heteroduplex stability is increased, which usually causes the K_M to fall toward its minimum. The benefit to the overall kinetic efficiency obtained by increasing binding domain length, however, is limited by the adverse effect it has on catalytic turnover (indicated by the k_{cat}), which occurs when the enzymes' increased affinity for the products slows down the catalytic cycle by reducing the rate of product release. In more recent investigation of this behavior in reactions where the substrate-binding domain length ranged between 4/4 (base length/arm) to 13/13, the maximum overall efficiency (k_{cat}/K_M) under physiological reaction conditions was found with an arm length of between 8 and 9 bp (5).

In addition to extraordinary cleavage activity and specificity, the 10–23 DNAzyme has a broad target range with its only substrate requirement being a purine–pyrimidine. This is ideal for target selection, as the more sites tested in long-folded mRNA, the greater the likelihood of finding highly accessible and cleavable sites *(13)*. It also means that DNAzymes can be targeted with greater flexibility to discrete sites such as those spanning polymorphisms or fusion transcripts produced as a consequence of chromosomal translocation. Despite the reported activity against any RY cleavage site, our early experiences with DNAzyme targeting RC dinucleotides indicated that these sequences were cleaved less efficiently than those containing RU were. This led us to exclude these cytosine sites in our search for DNAzymes with efficient gene-suppression activity *(13)*. To determine if there was a rational basis in our preference for RU cleavage sites over those consisting of RC, a systematic analysis of DNAzyme activity against various combination of RY-containing substrates was conducted. As each of these substrates was a derivative of a common ancestor, they all contained the same background sequence. From these experiments, it was found that there was a hierarchy of RY reactivity to the 10–23 DNAzyme, which appeared to follow the general scheme AU = GU ≥ GC >>AC.

In view of the relatively poor activity of RC cleavage sites (particularly AC), an attempt was made to modify the DNAzyme to improve its cleavage efficiency against these targets. One of the differences between RU and RC cleavage sites is the increased strength of the basepair interaction between the pyrimidine base in the substrate and its cognate purine in the binding domain of the DNAzyme. Interestingly, we found that various conservative substitutions that subtly disturb or weaken this interaction had a profoundly positive effect on the reaction rate and extent (Fig. 2). The enhancement of activity generated by these modifications has the potential to significantly broaden the utility of the 10–23 DNAzyme, particularly against RNA target sites that contain an AC dinucleotide core.

Most kinetic analysis of the 10–23 DNAzyme has been performed on molecules with symmetric RNA binding domains irrespective the contribution of each arm to the total thermodynamic stability of the enzyme-substrate complex. There is some evidence to suggest that the optimal design of a 10–23 DNAzyme for a given target site should take into account both the sequence and length of the individual binding arm to accommodate the differences in stability of their respective complexes with the substrate. Experiments with different length binding domains have shown that in some instances the rate of DNAzyme-catalyzed cleavage can be enhanced by asymmetric arm length truncation *(14)*. In the case of DNAzymes targeting the *c-myc* translation initiation region, we found that the

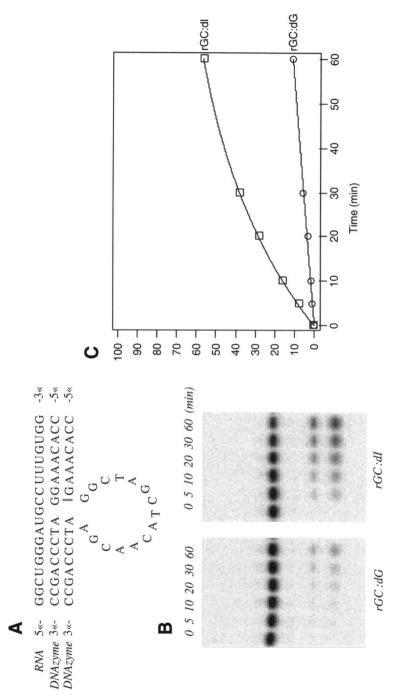

Fig. 2. Impact of inosine substitution on DNAzyme catalytic activity. (A) sequences of RNA substrate and designed DNAzymes. (B) in vitro cleavage activity of the wild type DNAzyme and inosine-substituted DNAzyme. (C) Reaction progress curves comparing the activity of rC-dG and rC-dI core substrate–DNAzyme pairs.

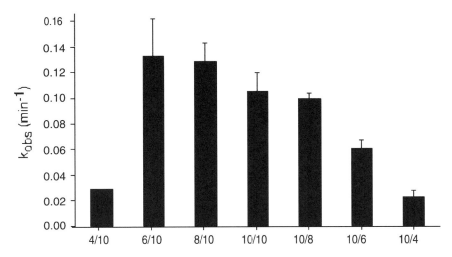

Fig. 3. Cleavage rate of asymmetric DNAzymes. k_{obs} was determined under the single turnover conditions.

observed reaction rate was highest in the molecule with a binding arm length ratio (5'/3' bp) of 6/10 (Fig. 3). This relative advantage derived by truncation of the binding domain on the 5' side of the catalytic domain was similar to that seen in the hammerhead ribozyme, which had an optimal length ratio (helix I/helix III), of 5/10 (15). The benefit of a shorter helix I in the ribozyme was attributed to a possible decrease in counterproductive interference between it and helix II. In the case of the DNA enzyme, which lacks the equivalent of a helix II, this effect is more likely related to the respective heteroduplex stability of each individual binding domain–substrate complex. In support of this argument, the hybridization free energy for the truncated 5' arm of the *c-myc*-cleaving DNAzyme was found to be unusually low, indicating that it was capable of generating more stability than expected for its size compared with the average duplex sequence.

3. TARGET SITE SELECTION

The design flexibility of the 10–23 DNAzyme is largely owing to its ability to bind a target RNA sequence via Watson–Crick basepair interactions. However, like other agents that function by hybridization with single-stranded RNA, the DNAzyme must compete with the targets own prevailing intramolecular basepairing, which can form stable secondary structures. Although most mRNA substrates provide a host of opportunities for DNAzyme cleavage, finding sites in the target RNA that are amenable to efficient hybridization and cleavage is usually a difficult and time-consuming task involving empirical testing of many

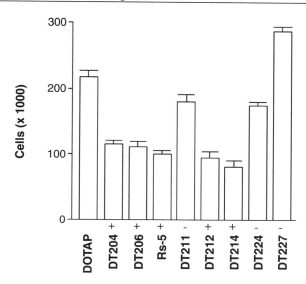

Fig. 4. Selected DNAzymes-mediated suppression of smooth muscle cell (SMC) proliferation. Five *c-myc*-cleaving DNAzymes selected (+) in a multiplex assay were compared with three DNAzymes that had no observable cleavage activity (–) in their ability
to suppress SMC proliferation. The level of growth suppression achieved by each treatment and the no DNAzyme control (DOTAP) was indicated by cell number. The sign
below each bar denoted the respective DNAzyme cleavage activity in vitro.

DNAzymes in long-folded RNA transcript in vitro. To streamline this process,
we developed a multiplex approach to target-site selection, which allowed the
simultaneous analysis of many different DNAzyme cleavage sites in a single
reaction *(13)*. This DNAzyme target-site selection strategy was used to identify
the most efficient cleavers of a full-length rat *c-myc* transcript. Some of the more
active molecules from 60 DNAzymes tested under multiplex conditions in vitro
were compared with less active cleavers in their ability to suppress rat smooth
muscle cell (SMC) proliferation (Fig. 4). As *c-myc* gene expression is closely
associated with proliferation in response to serum stimulation in this model, the
level of posttreatment growth could be used as an indicator of the anti-*c-myc*
activity. Gene suppression in this system was found to correlate with DNAzyme
activity in the multiplex cleavage assay, with the most efficient cleavers also
having the greatest effect on SMC proliferation. The multiplex assay was found
to be an effective screen for DNAzyme cleavage sites, because it could efficiently identify the molecules with high activity against a long- folded substrate
RNA. In addition to this application, the multiplex selection assay may also be
useful for identifying target-site accessibility for other RNA binding agents such
as antisense ONs and ribozymes.

3.1. Use of 10–23 DNAzyme for Nucleic Acid Sequence Detection

With the potential to bind any RNA sequence and cleave purine–pyrimidine junctions, the 10–23 DNA enzyme has an unprecedented target site flexibility. However, despite the enormous capacity to cleave different sequences, the actual substrate specificity of an individual DNAzyme with defined RNA-binding domains appears to be very high. This ability to discriminate is particularly important in biological applications where unwanted side reactions between the DNAzyme and some closely related or unrelated substrate could be very undesirable. We have also examined the specificity of the 10–23 DNAzyme by observing its ability to discriminate between sequences that differ by as little as a single nucleotide polymorphism *(9)*. In this experiment, reactions between DNAzyme and matching substrate sequences (derived from a polymorphic site in the L1 gene of six different clinically relevant human papilloma virus (HPV) types) were compared with reaction in the unmatched substrates. In each case only the perfectly matched type-specific DNAzymes were capable of achieving substantial cleavage of the corresponding substrate despite the similarity between the different sequences. In each of these studies the specificity of cleavage was examined with respect to binding domain–substrate interactions where some mismatches, particularly those producing a "wobble" pair, could be tolerated *(8,9)*. If, however, the difference between the target and nontarget substrate lies at the cleavage site, such that the purine–pyrimidine, R-Y, becomes R-R, Y-Y, or Y-R, then the DNAzyme would have no activity on the nontarget substrate.

Recently, a new strategy, called DzyNA, was proposed and demonstrated to use 10–23 DNAzymes to facilitate the detection of the products of in vitro amplification by polymerase chain reaction (PCR)*(16)*. In this assay, PCR is performed using a DzyNA primer that contains a target-specific sequence and the complementary (antisense) sequence of a 10–23 DNAzyme. Amplification of the target sequence will coincide with the generation of sense strand of the 10–23 DNAzymes, which can cleave a DNA/RNA chimeric reporter substrate, containing fluorescence resonance energy transfer fluorophores incorporated on either side of a DNAzyme cleavage site. In a real-time format, this assay proved to be a generic and flexible strategy that provides an alternative to other homogeneous amplification and detection systems, including the TaqMan™ and Molecular Beacon.

To demonstrate the potential clinical utility, DzyNA-PCR was used to estimate the concentrations of circulating K-*ras* DNA in the serum of patients with gastrointestinal malignancies *(16)*. Serum samples (5 μL) were estimated to contain between 10^3 and 10^4 copies of a single-copy gene (K-*ras*), indicating that the concentrations of circulating genomic DNA in these patients were in the range of 0.8–4 mg/L serum. DzyNA-PCR therefore allowed quantification of circulating DNA using only small amounts of the clinical specimens. The ability to detect tumor markers, such as microsatellite instability, aberrant methylation, or mutated oncogenes in serum or plasma may provide a new noninvasive tool for diagnosis, prognosis, and follow-up of cancer.

3.2. Use of 10–23 DNAzyme in Gene Suppression

The ability of the 10–23 DNAzyme to specifically cleave RNA with high efficiency under simulated physiological conditions has fueled expectation that this agent may have useful biological application in a gene-inactivation strategy. To explore this potential a number of groups have attempted to examine the activity of DNAzymes in biological systems *(13,17–28)*. In our laboratory we initiated experiments with DNAzymes targeting the viral sequences from the HPV 16 E6 and E7 genes; and in SMCs with DNAzymes targeting the *c-myc* gene *(13,17)*. These molecules designed against the translation initiation regions of *c-myc* and the HPV 16 E6 were optimized in terms of RNA-binding domain length through kinetic analysis of in vitro RNA cleavage reactions. To improve the stability of the DNAzyme ON to serum and intracellular nucleases while maintaining catalytic activity, a single 3'-terminal nucleotide inversion modification was introduced to the ONs during synthesis by the formation of a 3'–3' internucleotide linkage. After ensuring that the catalytic activity was preserved, the serum nuclease stability of the modified ONs was examined by incubation in 100% human serum. In this environment, ONs modified by 3' inversion were found to have a half-life of 24 h at 37°C compared with 2 h with the unmodified counterpart. The modified anti-E6 DNAzymes were cotransfected with an E6 gene expression vector into 3T3 cells with aid of the DOTAP transfection reagent. In this transient E6 expression system, the anti-E6 DNAzyme was found to substantially reduce the level of E6 mRNA compared with a nonactive ON with the same nucleotide composition (unpublished observations).

When proliferating rat SMCs were treated with anti *c-myc* DNAzymes targeting the translation initiation site, a range of molecules was found to suppress SMC proliferation after serum stimulation *(17)*. The molecular basis of this effect was supported by the level of both *c-myc* RNA in Northern blot analysis and metabolically labeled *c-myc* protein from immunoprecipitation. The dose–response of the lead molecule (Rs6) was very competitive with the best antisense counterpart with an IC_{50} around 50 nM. Surprisingly, the extent of biological effect on SMC proliferation with different length and modification analogues correlated with cleavage activity tests in both the full-length substrate and a short synthetic substrate in vitro *(17)*. This was exemplified by Rs6 (9/9 bp arms and 3' inversion) that demonstrated outstanding activity in all respects (Fig. 5).

Two different groups have examined the activity and specificity of DNAzymes in leukemic cells that contain the Philadelphia chromosome and express the *bcr-abl* fusion *(29,30)*. In both respects the DNAzymes compared favorably with previous work with hammerhead ribozymes and antisense ONs *(31)*. Intracellu-

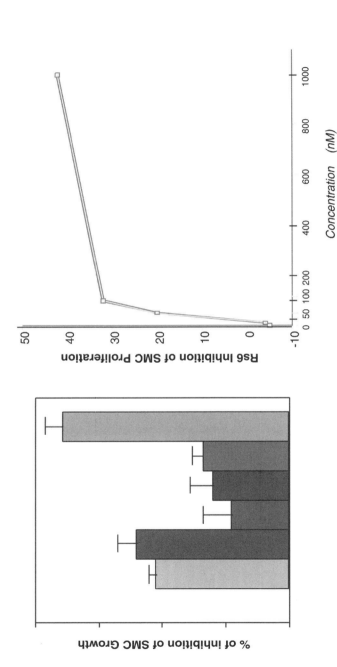

Fig. 5. (**A**) Growth-arrested smooth muscle cells (SMCs) were stimulated with 10% FBS-DME in the presence of $10\,\mu M$ anti-*c-myc* DNAzyme oligonucleotides or $10\,\mu M$ control oligonucleotide Rs8 (same arm sequences as Rs-6, with an inverted catalytic core sequence), or liposome alone (DOTAP). The data are displayed as mean ± SD. (**B**) Dose–response experiments for Rs-6 DNAzyme (9/9, 3' inversion) in SMCs. The data are expressed as % inhibition calculated from $(1 - \text{Rs6}/\text{Rs8})*100$.

lar activity of DNAzymes targeting the b2a2 splice junction was demonstrated with *bcr-abl*-luciferase and *abl*-luciferase reporter gene constructs in HeLa cells; and against endogenous *bcr-abl* and *abl* expressing BV173, H9 cells, respectively *(29)*. Similarly, DNAzymes also showed activity against the *bcr-abl* (b3a2) expression in K562 cells and CD34+ bone marrow cells from patients with chronic myelogenous leukemia *(30)*. The nuclease stability was enhanced in these molecules by capping the terminals with either two phosphorothioate linkages or by 2'-*O*-methyl modification of two terminal residues. Both of these modified DNAzymes were found to have sustained intracellular activity; however, in one study only the 2'-*O*-methyl modified molecules maintained specificity for the target *bcr-abl (29)*.

Another oncology target challenged recently with a DNAzyme is protein kinase C (PKC)-α . PKC-α DNAzymes were found to suppress the proliferation of various tissue culture lines and induce apoptosis *(24)*. The greatest serum stability was achieved in DNAzymes in which the catalytic domain pyrimidines as well as the entire binding domain were phosphorothioate modified. This stability, however, came with the expense of a 10-fold reduction in reaction rate.

Banerjea and coworkers have examined the activity of the 10–23 DNAzyme in an HIV model system. In this model, a luciferase reporter construct is used to indicate the extent of HIV-1 envelope-CD4-mediated cell fusion *(39)*. DNAzymes, which cleave the HIV *env* transcript, CCR5 chemokine receptor, and CXCR4 chemokine receptor, were all found to be potent inhibitors of fusion between CD-4 positive HeLa cells and HeLa cells expressing the HIV-1 envelope gene. In another group, DNAzymes directed to the conserved V3 loop of HIV *env* were capable of suppressing both viral replication (viral load/p24 antigen) and virus infection (single-cycle reporter system) *(29)*. In addition to HIV and its receptors, the 10–23 DNAzyme has also been shown to be active against viral mRNA targets from the hepatitis C and B, and was able to protect cells from infection with influenza A virus *(25–27)*.

The activity of the 10–23 DNAzyme has also been investigated against the *huntingtin* mRNA *(23)*. The mutant protein expressed from this transcript is thought to be the causative agent in Huntington's disease. The mutation responsible for this neurodegenerative disorder is derived from expansion of a CAG repeat, and though an ideal target, it was not susceptible to deoxyribonucleotide cleavage. However, despite the lack of activity in this area, DNAzymes specific for a number of other target sites were chosen on the basis of RNA secondary structure prediction. Two of these DNAzymes demonstrated substantial activity against the *huntingtin* transcript in vitro and protein in HEK-293 cells cotransfected with the *huntingtin* gene. Interestingly, the intracellular activity of these two DNAzymes when used together (at half the active concentration) was synergistic, such that the overall suppression gene expression was greater than when tested individually.

A DNAzyme targeting the transcription factor Egr-1 has been shown to inhibit SMC proliferation in culture and neointima formation in the rat carotid artery damaged by ligation injury or balloon angioplasty *(21)*. Suppression of Egr-1 was also monitored at the RNA and protein level in treated SMCs by Northern and Western blot analysis, respectively. This was the first evidence of DNAzyme efficacy in vivo, and, furthermore, the activity displayed by this anti-Egr-1 molecule could potentially find application in various forms of cardiovascular disease such as restenosis.

3.3. Use of DNAzyme in Target Validation

The application of genomics is currently one of the central issues in pharmaceutical drug discovery. Although the Human Genome Project is officially only 8 yr old, many consider that it has already entered the "postgenomics" era. For pharmaceutical research and development, this means that attention is turning toward the biological characterization of the thousands of new genes that are catalogued in databases. Therefore, determining the function of novel genes identified by the Human Genome Project is a key challenge in future drug discovery and development efforts.

For efficient validation of new genes, the expression pattern of the candidate genes within the whole body, and specifically within the organ or tissue of interest, can be used as the first level of understanding. Secondary testing, such as functional expression and knockdown studies, and bioinformatic analysis of full-length cDNAs, is then used according to the particular gene under investigation. If the gene(s) of interest are found to be a multitype gene family and endogenously expressed in cultured cells, consideration should be given to examining the effects of knockdown studies. Obviously, the technology that is required for this purpose needs to be specific but broadly applicable, and it must have the ability to be applied with only limited information on the target. DNAzyme technology may represent one of the ideal choices for gene suppression because it has a moderate-throughput capacity and acts in a sequence-specific way. This capacity for highly flexible binding and discrimination of nucleic acid substrates by virtue of Watson–Crick interactions will enable DNAzymes to facilitate gene-type specific reactions for gene function validation with very high precision.

4. CONCLUSION

RNA is clearly an attractive target for biological and therapeutic manipulation. In the cellular machinery it usually appears as a dynamic intermediate between the genetic information encoded by DNA and the functional protein units. Although the structural and functional complexity and diversity of proteins make them relatively easy targets for small molecule inhibitors, it is difficult to predict (for different proteins) which ones will be effective and specific. The relative structural homogeneity of RNA, although difficult to specifically inhibit with traditional small molecules drugs, provides the opportunity for a generic approach to targeting through its sequence. This form of digital or information-level, recognition is essentially achievable with nucleic acid compounds because of their ability to hybridize in a sequence-dependent manner with their complementary targets. This in essence provides a universal system for rational sequence-specific targeting, drawing on information that is easily obtainable—the genome—rather than more elusive protein structure–function data. Appealing as this concept seems, nucleic acid reagents have not quite lived up to expectation. The main problem lies in two different aspects of target accessibility. First, RNA is an intracellular target and hence is protected to a large extent from the influence of large polyanionic ONs present in the extracellular fluid. Second, for those molecules that do colocalize with their target, to bind it they may encounter another layer of accessibility problems generated by the target RNA's own intramolecular basepairing.

Recent developments in catalytic DNA provide an opportunity to couple the RNA cleavage activity of ribozymes with simple and robust chemistry of the ON. These DNAzymes have shown themselves to be capable of efficient gene suppression in a number of biological systems in vitro and in vivo. This new class of molecule, although showing a lot of promise, still consists of nucleic acid and therefore must overcome many of the same obstacles experienced by other reagents of this type. Methodology for finding optimal DNAzyme cleavage sites that correspond to regions of high RNA accessibility in vitro has been established and should help streamline the process of target site selection. To increase the bioactive intracellular concentration of DNAzymes, a range of formulations are being explored that enhance delivery of ONs to both the cytoplasm and nucleus. These delivery protocols are allowing DNAzymes to access their targets both in vitro culture systems and in vivo model systems with potential applications in gene function discovery, target validation, and therapeutics. Success in these areas with DNAzymes (as with other nucleic-acid-based approaches) is linked with technology that facilitates delivery.

REFERENCES

1. Crooke, ST. Molecular mechanisms of antisense drugs. Antisense Nucleic Acid Drug Dev 1998; 8:133.
2. Symons RH. Ribozymes. Curr Opin Struct Biol 1994; 4:322.
3. Breaker RR, Joyce GF. A DNA enzyme that cleaves RNA. Chem Biol 1994; 1:223–229.
4. Breaker RR, Joyce GF. A DNA enzyme with Mg (2+)-dependent RNA phosphoesterase activity. Chem Biol 1995; 2:655–660.
5. Santoro SW, Joyce GF. A general purpose RNA-cleaving DNA enzyme. Proc Natl Acad Sci USA 1997; 94:4262–4266.
6. Breaker RR. DNA Enzymes. Nat Biotech 1997; 15:427–431.
7. Li Y, Breaker RR. Deoxyribozymes: new players in the ancient game of biocatalysis. Curr Opin Struct Biol 1999; 9:315–323.

8. Santoro SW, Joyce GF. Mechanism and utility of an RNA-cleaving DNA enzyme. Biochemistry 1998; 37:13330–13342.

9. Cairns MJ, King A, Sun LQ. Nucleic acid mutation analysis using catalytic DNA. Nucleic Acids Res 2000; 28:e9.

10. Sugimoto N, Nakano S, Katoh M, et al. Thermodynamic parameters to predict stability of RNA/DNA hybrid duplexes. Biochemistry 1995; 34:11211–11216.

11. Ratmeyer L, Vinayak R, Zhong YY, Zon G, Wilson WD. Sequence specific thermodynamic and structural properties for DNA–RNA duplexes. Biochemistry 1994; 33:5298–530412. Gyi JI, Lane AN, Conn GL, Brown T. Solution structures of DNA–RNA hybrids with purine-rich and pyrimidine rich strands: Comparison with homologous DNA and RNA duplexes. Biochemistry 1998; 37:73–80

12. Gyi JL, Lane AN, Conn GL, Brown T. Solution structures of DNA•RNA hybrids with purine-rich and pyrimidine rich strands: Comparison with homologous DNA and RNA duplexes. Biochemistry 1998;37:73–80.

13. Cairns MJ, Hopkins TM, Witherington C, Wang L, Sun LQ. Target site selection for an RNA-cleaving catalytic DNA. Nat Biotech 1999; 17:480–486.

14. Cairns MJ, Hopkins TM, Witherington C, Sun LQ. The influence of arm length asymmetry and base substitution on the activity of the 10–23 DNA enzyme. Antisense Nucleic Acid Drug Dev. 2000; 10:323–332.

15. Hendry P, McCall M J. Unexpected anisotropy in substrate cleavage rates by asymmetric hammerhead ribozymes. Nucleic Acids Res 1996; 24:2679–2684.

16. Todd AV, Fuery CJ, Impey HL, Applegate TL, Haughton MA. DzyNA-PCR: use of DNAzymes to detect and quantify nucleic acid sequences in a real-time fluorescent format. Clin Chem. 2000; 46: 625–630.

17. Sun LQ, Cairns MJ, Gerlach WL, Witherington C, Wang L, King A. Suppression of smooth muscle cell proliferation by a c-myc RNA-cleaving deoxyribozyme. J Biol Chem 1999; 274:17236–17241.

18. Dash BC, Harikrishnan TA, Goila R, et al. Targeted cleavage of HIV-1 envelope gene by a DNA enzyme and inhibition of HIV-1 envelope-CD4 mediated cell fusion. FEBS Lett 1998; 431:395–399.

19. Zhang X, Xu Y, Ling H, Hattori T. Inhibition of infection of incoming HIV-1 virus by RNA-cleaving DNA enzyme. FEBS Lett 1999; 458:151–156.

20. Goila R, Banerjea AC. Sequence specific cleavage of the HIV-1 coreceptor CCR5 gene by a hammerhead ribozyme and a DNA-enzyme: inhibition of the coreceptor function by DNA-enzyme. FEBS Lett 1998; 436:233–238.

21. Santiago FS, Kavurma MM, Lowe HC, et al. New DNA enzyme targeting Egr-1 mRNA inhibits vascular smooth muscle proliferation and regrowth after injury. Nat Med 1999; 5:1264–1269.

22. Basu S, Sriram B, Goila R, Banerjea AC. Targeted cleavage of HIV-1 coreceptor-CXCR-4 by RNA-cleaving DNA-enzyme: inhibition of coreceptor function. Antiviral Res. 2000; 46:125–134.

23. Yen L, Strittmatter SM, Kalb RG. Sequence-specific cleavage of Huntington mRNA by catalytic DNA. Ann Neurol 1999; 46:366–373.

24. Sioud M, Leirdal M. Design of nuclease resistant protein kinase calpha DNA enzymes with potential therapeutic application. J Mol Biol. 2000; 296:937–947.

25. Oketani M, Asahina Y, Wu CH, Wu GY. Inhibition of hepatitis C virus-directed gene expression by a DNA ribonuclease. J Hepatol. 1999; 31:628–634.

26. Goila R, Banerjea AC. Inhibition of hepatitis B virus X gene expression by novel DNA enzymes. Biochem J. 2001; 353(Pt 3):701–708.

27. Toyoda T, Imamura Y, Takaku H, et al. Inhibition of influenza virus replication in cultured cells by RNA-cleaving DNA enzyme. FEBS Lett. 2000; 48:113–116.

28. Liu C, Cheng R, Sun LQ, Tien P. Suppression of platelet-type 12-lipoxygenase activity in human erythroleukemia cells by an RNA-cleaving DNAzyme. Biochem Biophys Res Commun. 2001; 284:1077–1082.
29. Warashina M, Kuwabara T, Nakamatsu, Y, Taira K. Extremely high and specific activity of DNA enzymes in cells with a Philadelphia chromosome. Chem Biol 1999; 6:237–250.
30. Wu Y, Yu L, McMahon R, Rossi JJ, Forman SJ, Snyder DS. Inhibition of bcr-abl oncogene expression by novel deoxyribozymes (DNAzymes). Hum Gene Ther 1999; 10:2847–2857.
31. Gewirtz AM, Sokol DL, Ratajczak MZ. Nucleic acid therapeutics: state of the art and future prospects. Blood 1998; 92:712–736.

6 Targeted Destruction of Small, Stable RNAs

Principles Applicable to Antisense Therapies

David A. Dunbar, PhD
and Susan J. Baserga, MD, PhD

1. INTRODUCTION

Antisense deoxyoligonucleotides have been used for some time as tools for the targeted destruction of specific RNA molecules. Although antisense oligonucleotides (ONs) were originally used to destroy mRNAs in order to reveal the function of specific proteins, their use has logically been extended to therapy for diseases that result from the unwanted expression of specific proteins, as in cancer. However, choosing the ON to target mRNAs in these cases has largely been empirical. Some important information regarding the choice of ON can be gleaned from numerous studies that have used antisense ONs to probe the function of small nuclear and small nucleolar RNAs (snRNAs and snoRNAs, respectively). When an ON is designed to target an mRNA, the RNA structure and the

From: *Cancer Drug Discovery and Development:*
Nucleic Acid Therapeutics in Cancer
Edited by: A. M. Gewirtz © Humana Press Inc., Totowa, NJ

areas where the mRNA-associated proteins bind are largely unknown. In contrast, the structure of small RNAs and the proteins that bind to them are generally known, lending a rational approach to antisense ON design. Therefore, the study of the function of small RNAs, both in vivo and in vitro, may provide crucial insight for developing antisense therapies.

When complexed with their associated proteins, snRNAs and snoRNAs become ribonucleoproteins (snRNPs and snoRNPs). These two RNPs have different subcellular localizations and different functions: snRNPs (U1, U2, U4, U5, and U6) splice pre-mRNAs in the nucleoplasm, and snoRNPs are required for cleavage and modification of pre-rRNAs in the nucleolus. Most small RNAs are only 70–300 nucleotides in length, and their secondary structure, in the presence and absence of protein components, can be determined by chemical and enzymatic means and by phylogenetic comparisons.

Likewise, the portions of the small RNAs covered with protein can be ascertained. Because small RNA secondary structures and protein binding sites can be determined, the function of these RNPs has been established by depletion of the snoRNAs via antisense ON targeting.

2. ON-DIRECTED RNASE H-MEDIATED RNA CLEAVAGE IN HELA CELL EXTRACTS

ONs were first used to target the snRNPs, U1 and U2, in cell-free extracts to determine their roles in pre-mRNA splicing. This was first accomplished by Kramer et al. *(1)* in a HeLa cell nuclear extract, with an ON directed to the first eight nucleotides of the U1 snRNA. Site-directed cleavage of this portion of the RNA was carried out with exogenously added RNase H in the presence of the deoxyoligonucleotide. RNase H cleaves the RNA component of the RNA:DNA hybrid at the site of hybridization *(2)*. These authors reasoned that the 5' end of the U1 snRNA would be accessible to the oligonucleotide because it was this portion of U1 snRNA that was available for binding to the 5' splice site of a mRNA precursor through complementary basepairing. Subsequently, Black et al. *(3)* and Krainer and Maniatis *(4)* performed similar studies using HeLa cell extracts to demonstrate that the U1 and the U2 snRNAs were involved in splicing. In Black et al. only those antisense ONs targeted to the proposed single-stranded regions of the U2 snRNA were successful in cleavage upon the addition of exogenous RNase H. However, not all the ONs targeted to proposed single-stranded regions of the U2 snRNA led to RNA cleavage after RNase H addition, suggesting that there must be additional parameters required. As these authors point out, ON-mediated RNase H digestion can only be successful if the targeted sequence is available for basepairing (single-stranded), and if it is accessible to RNase H. Therefore, both snRNP-associated proteins and RNA secondary structure may interfere with ON targeting.

Subsequently, ON-mediated RNase H cleavage was carried out to examine whether the U4 and U6 snRNAs were required for pre-mRNA splicing. Black and Steitz *(5)* were able to cleave both U4 and U6 snRNAs in HeLa nuclear extracts with antisense ONs directed toward single-stranded regions not bound by proteins. They then went on to show that U4 and U6 are required for pre-mRNA splicing. In contrast, Berget and Robberson *(6)*, who also examined the effect of U4 snoRNA cleavage, were not able to find any of three ONs that would induce RNase H-mediated cleavage of U6. Interestingly, one of their ONs (nt 43–55), which yielded negative results overlaps with one used by Black and Steitz (nt 43–60) that did give partial cleavage (and an effect on pre-mRNA splicing), indicating that length of complementarity may also play a role. Berget and Robberson then showed that U1, U2, and U4 are required for pre-mRNA splicing but not for polyadenylation. They found no ONs that were able to cleave the U5 snRNA in HeLa cell extracts in the presence of RNase H.

3. IN VIVO ON-TARGETED RNASE H-MEDIATED SNRNA AND SNORNA CLEAVAGE

Antisense ONs have also been used to destroy snRNAs in *Xenopus* oocytes, not only to reveal their role in pre-mRNA splicing but also to test the function of different portions of the small RNAs. This can be done because microinjected small RNAs assemble with their *Xenopus* protein components. Pan and Prives *(7,8)* depleted the U1 and U2 snRNAs by microinjection of antisense DNA ONs into *Xenopus* oocyte nuclei and demonstrated that pre-mRNA splicing was blocked. Presumably, RNA degradation was carried out by endogenous RNase H (Fig. 1) *(9)*. The choice of oligonucleotide to be microinjected was based on ONs successfully used by others in HeLa cell extracts. Efficient splicing could be restored by subsequent microinjection of HeLa U1 and U2 snRNAs. This provides convincing genetic evidence that the observed defect in pre-mRNA splicing is due to the degradation of these specific RNAs. This kind of "rescue" experiment is essential for interpretation of in vivo experiments because the injected ONs may have multiple, unanticipated targets (see "Unexpected snoRNA targets" later in this chapter). Mattaj and colleagues *(10–12)* have used this approach to dissect the functional domains of the U1, U2, U4, and U6 snRNAs.

The U3 snoRNA was the first snoRNA to be disrupted by injection of antisense ONs into *Xenopus* oocytes *(13)*. Microinjection of an oligonucleotide complementary to U3 snoRNA nts 61–75 was able to deplete 97% of the U3 snoRNA after repeated injection. However, although changes in the levels of some pre-rRNA intermediates were observed, leading to the conclusion that pre-rRNA processing was affected, levels of the mature processed pre-rRNAs were not affected. Investigation of whether restoration of normal levels of the U3 snoRNA by microinjection would return the levels of processing precursors to normal was not carried out.

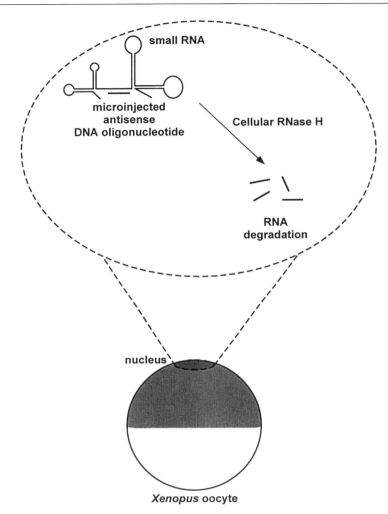

Fig. 1. Depletion of small RNAs in *Xenopus* oocytes by antisense DNA ONs. The targeted small RNAs, which are complexed with proteins as ribonucleoproteins, are found in the nuclear or nucleolar compartments. Short, antisense DNA ONs are microinjected in either the cytoplasm or nucleus. Provided that the targeted sequence is single-stranded and accessible to the oligonucleotide, small RNA-oligonucleotide basepairing occurs, triggering the endogenous RNase H. Degradation of the RNA and snRNP/snoRNP disruption therefore results.

More recent experiments where U3 was depleted by microinjection of different ONs revealed that normal levels of processing intermediates and, in this case, mature 18S rRNA could be restored by microinjection of U3 *(14)*.

Similarly, microinjection of ONs directed against the U8 snoRNA revealed that it was required for processing of precursors to the 5.8S and 28S large ribosomal subunit rRNAs. Three ONs were tested for their ability to deplete the U8 snoRNA based on its predicted secondary structure; two were able to deplete U8 almost completely after two cytoplasmic injections. Upon depletion of U8, mature 5.8S and 28S rRNAs were absent and accumulation of aberrant precursors was seen. In this case, microinjection of U8 snoRNA restored pre-rRNA processing, indicating that the observed RNA processing defect was due to the absence of U8. Likewise, depletion of the U22 snoRNA by microinjection of either of 2 ONs into the cytoplasm of *Xenopus* oocytes interfered with processing of pre-18S rRNAs *(15)*. Again, normal pre-rRNA processing was restored by microinjection of the U22 snoRNA.

Many of the approx 200 snoRNAs in metazoan cells are not required for pre-rRNA cleavage but instead play a role in pre-rRNA modification reviewed in *(16)*. snoRNAs are required for both 2' -*O*-ribose methylation and for pseudouridylation of the pre-rRNA. Depletion of one of the putative methylation guide snoRNAs, U25, by cytoplasmic microinjection of an antisense oligonucleotide, led to loss of methylation at G1448 in the 18S rRNA *(17)*. Microinjection of either human or *Xenopus* U25 snoRNA restored methylation. Similarly, injection of two antisense ONs complementary to the U26 snoRNA led to complete degradation of U26 and loss of methylation at A394 in the 28S rRNA *(18)*. For depletion of the U14 snoRNA, coinjection of two nonoverlapping antisense ONs resulted in more efficient depletion than injection of either one alone *(19)*.

4. UNEXPECTED MULTIPLE SNORNA TARGETS: PITFALLS FOR THERAPEUTICS

Our studies on the function of the U18 snoRNA illuminated the pitfalls of targeting RNAs for depletion in vivo *(20)*. Four ONs were tested for their ability to deplete the U18 snoRNA; three of the four successfully depleted U18 when injected (Fig. 2). However, subsequent analysis of pre-rRNA processing gave a surprising result. Of the three ONs that depleted U18, only injection of oligo 18.1 caused a defect in pre-18S rRNA processing. In addition, one of them that did not deplete U18, 18.3, produced a partial defect in pre-rRNA processing. Careful sleuthing indicated that injection of the 18.1 oligonucleotide, in addition to depleting the U18 snoRNA, also depleted the U22 snoRNA (Fig. 2). The U22 snoRNA had previously been shown to be required for pre-18S rRNA processing *(15)*. Sequence inspection indicated that targeting of the U22 snoRNA with the 18.1 oligonucleotide occurred because of six nucleotides of complementarity, within an accessible region in U22, indicating that in vivo six nucleotides of

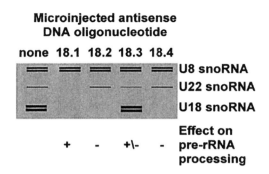

Fig. 2. Antisense DNA oligonucleotides (ONs) designed to be specific can have multiple RNA targets. Antisense DNA ONs designed to target U18 (18.1–18.4) were injected into *Xenopus* oocytes. To check for depletion, RNA was harvested 24 h postinjection and analyzed for the presence of the U8, U22 and U18 snoRNAs by Northern blots. There are two forms of U8 in *Xenopus* oocytes that differ in length (Christopher Chang and Susan Baserga, unpublished). Pre-rRNA processing was analyzed 24 h postinjection. This schematic was drawn from results presented in *20*.

complementarity is sufficient to activate RNase H. Injection of the 18.3 oligonucleotide depletes U22 incompletely, accounting for the partial defect in pre-rRNA processing. The 18.3 oligonucleotide also shares the same six nucleotides of complementarity with the U22 snoRNA; however, it occurs in the middle of the oligonucleotide, instead of at one of the ends like in the 18.1 oligonucleotide. This indicates that the position of the complementarity is also important for RNase H-mediated snoRNA depletion. We proved the effect on pre-rRNA processing was due to depletion of U22 because the processing defect could be restored by microinjection of the U22 snoRNA, but not by microinjection of the U18 snoRNA. Therefore our microinjected ONs, although carefully chosen to be specific for targeted cleavage of the U18 snoRNA, were also able to cleave another snoRNA.

Depletion of the "wrong" RNA also occurred in experiments designed to target the MRP RNA. Experiments were designed to test the function of the MRP RNA, at that time a small RNA of unknown nucleolar function, in pre-rRNA processing. To examine its function, we attempted to deplete the *Xenopus* MRP *(21)* via injection of antisense ONs. Although we used a series of ONs that would have covered the entire RNA, we were not successful. It is now known that the MRP RNA is associated with a number of proteins *(22)*, likely rendering the RNA inaccessible to the ONs. However, we did serendipitously discover that one of the tested ONs was successful at depleting a U8 snoRNA variants (unpublished). Again, here is an example where a specific, complementary oligonucleotide targeted an RNA distinct from that for which it was designed.

5. CONCLUSIONS

Our work in *Xenopus* oocytes indicates that targeting specific RNA molecules with anti-sense ONs can inadvertently target other RNA molecules as well. For experiments designed to answer questions about function this result emphasizes the importance of the genetic "rescue" experiment. For use of antisense ONs in therapeutics, it points out that one of the potential problems may be unanticipated targeting of other mRNAs.

REFERENCES

1. Kramer A, Keller W, Appel B, Luhrmann R. The 5' terminus of the RNA moiety of U1 small nuclear ribonucleoprotein particles is required for the splicing of messenger RNA precursors. Cell 1984; 38:299–307.
2. Donis-Keller H. Site specific enzymatic cleavage of RNA. Nuc Acids Res 1979; 7:179–192.
3. Black DL, Chabot B, Steitz JA. U2 as well as U1 small nuclear ribonucleoproteins are involved in premessenger RNA splicing. Cell 1985; 42:737–750.
4. Krainer AR, Maniatis T. Multiple factors including the small nuclear ribonucleoproteins U1 and U2 are necessary for pre-mRNA splicing in vitro. Cell 1985; 42:725–736.
5. Black DL, Steitz JA. Pre-mRNA splicing in vitro requires intact U4/U6 small nuclear ribonucleoprotein. Cell 1986; 46:697–704.
6. Berget SM, Robberson BL. U1, U2 and U4/U6 small nuclear ribonucleoproteins are required for in vitro splicing but not polyadenylation. Cell 1986; 46:691–696.
7. Pan ZQ, Prives C. Assembly of functional U1 and U2 human-amphibian hybrid snRNPs in Xenopus laevis oocytes. Science 1988; 241:1328–1331.
8. Pan ZQ, Prives C. U2 snRNA sequences that bind U2-specific proteins are dispensable for the function of the U2 snRNP in splicing. Genes Dev 1989; 3:1887–1898.
9. Rebagliati MR, Melton D. Antisense RNA injections in fertilized frog eggs reveal an RNA duplex unwinding activity. Cell 1987; 48:599–605.
10. Hamm J, Dathan NA, Mattaj IW. Functional analysis of mutant Xenopus U2 snRNAs. Cell 1989; 59:159–169.
11. Hamm J, Dathan NA, Scherly D, Mattaj IW. Multiple domains of U1 snRNA, including U1 specific protein binding sites, are required for splicing. EMBO Journal 1990; 9:1237–1244.
12. Vankan P, McGuigan C, Mattaj IW. Domains of U4 and U6 snRNAs required for snRNP assembly and splicing complementation in Xenopus oocytes. EMBO J 1990; 9:3397–3404.
13. Savino R, Gerbi SA. In vivo disruption of Xenopus U3 snRNA affects ribosomal RNA processing. EMBO J 1990; 9:2299–2308.
14. Borovjagin AV, Gerbi SA. U3 small nucleolar RNA is essential for cleavage at sites 1, 2 and 3 in pre-rRNA and determines which rRNA processing pathway is taken in Xenopus oocytes. J Mol Biol 1999; 286:1347–1363.
15. Tycowski KT, Shu MD, Steitz JA. Requirement for intron-encoded U22 small nucleolar RNA in 18S ribosomal RNA processing. Science 1994; 266:1558–1561.
16. Smith CM, Steitz JA. Sno storm in the nucleolus: new roles for myriad small RNPs. Cell 1997; 89:669–672.
17. Tycowski KT, Smith CM, Shu MD, Steitz JA. A small nucleolar RNA requirement for site-specific ribose methylation of rRNA in Xenopus. Proc. Natl. Acad. Sci. USA 1996; 93:14480–14485.

18. Yu YT, Shu MD, Steitz JA. A new method for detecting sites of 2' -O-methylation in RNA molecules. RNA 1997; 3:324–351.

19. Dunbar DA, Baserga SJ. The U14 snoRNA is required for 2' -O-methylation of the pre-18S rRNA in Xenopus oocytes. RNA 1998; 4:195–204.

20. Dunbar DA, Ware VC, Baserga SJ. The U18 snRNA is not essential for pre-rRNA processing in Xenopus laevis. RNA 1996; 2:324–333.

21. Bennett JL, Jeong-Yu S, Clayton DA. Characterization of a Xenopus laevis ribonucleoprotein endoribonuclease. J Biol Chem 1992; 267:21765–21772.

22. Chamberlain JR, Lee Y, Lane WS, Engelke DR. Purification and characterization of the nuclear RNase P holoenzyme complex reveals extensive subunit overlap with RNase MRP. Genes Dev. 1998; 12:1678–1690.

7

Mechanism of Action of Antisense RNA in Eukaryotic Cells

Zuo Zhang, PhD
and Gordon G. Carmichael, PhD

CONTENTS

For many years, an appealing strategy to target the inhibition of expression of specific cellular or viral genes has been to express within cells RNA transcripts that have the potential to form duplex RNA hybrids with their target messages *(1)*. Although there are numerous examples in the literature of the successful application of antisense strategy, the many failures and frustrations have been less well documented. Recent work from a number of laboratories, and from a number of different experimental directions, has begun to provide a molecular framework for understanding how antisense RNA works within cells. Understanding these "rules" for antisense RNA holds the promise to aid in the future design and implementation of more effective antisense approaches. In this chapter we will discuss some of the current knowledge about how antisense RNA works. It has become apparent in the past several years that the formation of double-stranded RNA (dsRNA), triggers a variety of cellular effects that depend not only on the length of the RNA duplex, but also on its intracellular location and on the cell type *(1)*. These effects include activation of the protein kinase (PKR) and RNase L pathways, interferon responses, covalent modification of dsRNAs, and regulation of specific gene expression such as genomic imprinting. Most recently, the discovery of the remarkable phenomenon of dsRNA-induced RNA interference (RNAi) in cells of higher eukaryotes has become one of the great breakthroughs in studying the regulation of gene expression *(2–6)*.

From: *Cancer Drug Discovery and Development:*
Nucleic Acid Therapeutics in Cancer
Edited by: A. M. Gewirtz © Humana Press Inc., Totowa, NJ

1. DSRNA ACTION IN THE CYTOPLASM

1.1. Nonspecific and Global Inhibition: Interferon, PKR, RNase L, Apoptosis

In mammalian cells, cytoplasmic dsRNA can trigger a profound physiological reaction, which is primarily an antiviral defense pathway and which is dsRNA sequence-independent *(1,7)*. This pathway is summarized in Fig. 1. Most viral infections or other dsRNAs generated in cytoplasm induce type I interferons (IFNs), including IFN-α and IFN-β. IFNs are multifunctional cytokines that modulate host immunological functions and can inhibit tumor cell growth and virus multiplication *(7,8)*. After synthesis, IFNs are secreted to extracellular compartment, function on neighboring cells as paracrine cytokines, and induce IFN-stimulated genes (ISGs) *(9)*. The dsRNA-activated serine/threonine PKR plays a central role in cytoplasmic dsRNA activity *(10–12)*. IFNs are also involved in the activation of the PKR pathway *(13)*. Mammalian cells normally contain basal levels of PKR, but in an unphosphorylated, inactive form. When dsRNA is introduced into cytoplasm, PKR binds to and is activated by the activator dsRNA, which induces dimerization and autophosphorylation *(14–16)*. PKR can be activated by low concentrations of dsRNA, while being inhibited by higher dsRNA concentrations. Activated PKR can phosphorylate IκB *(17)*, which causes the release of the transcription factor NFκB to translocate to the nucleus and activates the expression of genes having NFκB binding sites, including the IFN-β gene. The translation factor eIF2a is another substrate phosphorylated by active PKR *(18)*. eIF2a phosphorylation results the global down-regulation of protein synthesis and gene expression *(19)*.

Cytoplasmic dsRNA and IFNs also activate the 2', 5'-adenylate synthase (AS)/RNase L pathway so that 2',5'-AS polymerizes ATP and other nucleotides in 2',5' linkage *(20–22)*. These 2',5' oligoadenylates then activate the ribonuclease RNase L *(23)*, which can cleave both cellular and viral RNAs and can also induce apoptosis *(24,25)*. Through a combination of the IFN, PKR, and RNase L pathways, cytoplasmic dsRNA normally causes a nonspecific inhibition of gene expression and complex cellular effects. As most cytoplasmic dsRNAs derive from viral infections, these pathways appear to serve primarily as host antiviral responses.

1.2. Specific Inhibition of Gene Expression: RNA Interference (RNAi)

RNAi was first discovered in *C. elegans* by Fire and Mello *(26)*, who originally showed that the mixture of sense and antisense strands silenced expression of a target gene much more efficiently than either strand alone. This phenomenon has also been observed in *Drosophila* and plants, and most recently in mouse

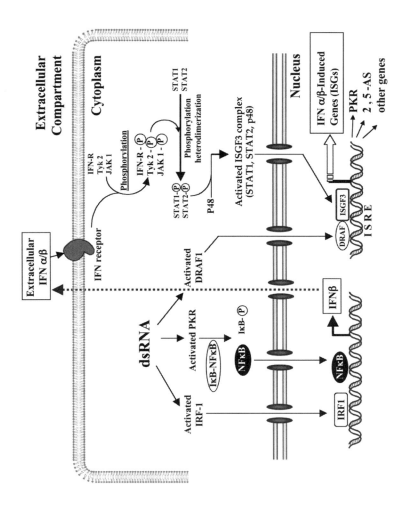

Fig. 1. Signaling pathways of IFNα, IFNβ and long cytoplasmic dsRNA. The major known pathways of signaling by cytoplasmic dsRNA and IFNα/β are shown. dsRNA directly activates PKR, IRF-1, and DRAF1. PKR phosphorylates IκB, which in turn leads to the nuclear localization of the transcription factor NFκB. IRF-1 and NFκB activate the IFN-β promoter, while DRAF1 can activate IFNα/β-induced genes (ISGs). IFN-β is secreted from cells (dashed arrow), then binds to IFN receptors, leading to the activation of the signal transduction pathway shown that itself stimulates the expression of ISGs.

91

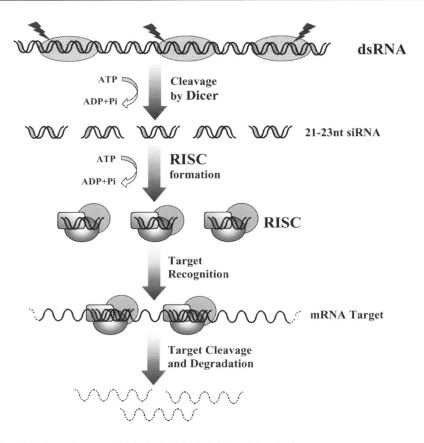

Fig. 2. RNA interference (RNAi). RNAi is initiated by the input trigger dsRNA, which is processed into 21-23 nucleotide guide sequences (siRNA) by a specific dsRNA endo-nuclease, Dicer. One strand of the siRNAs is incorporated into a nuclease complex, called the RNA-induced silencing complex (RISC). RISC acts to degrade the target mRNA recognized by siRNA through basepairing interactions. Cleavage by Dicer and the RISC formation are ATP-dependent.

embryos and cultured mammalian cells *(27–32)*. RNAi is a process by which the trigger dsRNA targets the specific degradation of homologous mRNA and thus silences its expression. Intensive biochemical and genetic studies on RNAi have been carried out over the past several years, and a great deal has been learned about the mechanistic basis of RNAi action *(2–6)* and is summarized in Fig. 2.

Although it has not been directly proved in vivo, RNAi most likely operates in the cytoplasm. In lower eukaryotes, a long dsRNA trigger is first processed by a multidomain RNase-III-like enzyme, Dicer, to 21–23 nt "short interfering RNAs" (siRNAs) *(27,33)*. siRNAs are then incorporated into the RNA-induced silencing complex (RISC), which targets to the homologous mRNA via Watson–Crick basepairing *(34)*. The target mRNA is cleaved and degraded by an unknown mechanism. By immunofluorescence, Dicer has been shown to localize to the cytoplasm of embryonal carcinoma cells and HeLa cells *(35)*. Long dsRNA can successfully induce RNAi in *C. elegans* and *Drosophila* cells, but this application is severely limited in mammalian cells because of the dominant pathway activated by dsRNA (the IFN, PKR, RNase L pathway discussed earlier) *(5,29,30)*. Exposing long dsRNA of any sequence to mammalian cells usually induces a nonspecific global shutdown of all gene expression *(1)*. Studies from Tuschl group, in which short siRNAs (21–22 nt) were introduced into cultured mammalian cells, indicated that specific inhibition of expression of target genes can be obtained without activating the nonspecific pathway. This work has paved the way to applying RNAi to specific silencing gene expression in mammalian cells *(29)*. In fact, this approach has recently been reported to be successful in rendering cells resistant to viral infection *(36)*.

Although the inhibition mediated by siRNA was not as efficient as by long dsRNA in *C. elegans* or *Drosophila* cells, it still made it promising for applying RNAi in mammalian cells *(29)*. As siRNA can only cover a small part of the target sequence, it is generally recommended to choose several sets of siRNAs, which cover different sequences, to obtain optimal inhibition. Recent work by Hannon and colleagues *(30)* has shown that in some cultured murine cells, such as embryonic cells and some mouse somatic cells, gene expression can be specifically silenced upon treatment with even long dsRNA. More importantly, stable sequence-specific silencing can be observed by enforcing endogenous expression of long RNA hairpins, which creates permanent cell lines with a desired loss-of-function phenotype. Other groups also showed that RNAi response can be induced effectively by long dsRNA in nondifferentiated mouse cells grown in culture *(35)*. These special cell lines presumably lack the nonspecific pathway to dsRNA, such as IFN and PKR *(30)*. Inhibition of endogenous PKR activity can enhance the specific silencing of gene expression, and reduce the nonspecific silencing, which suggests the usually dominant role of PKR and IFN pathway in host response to cytoplasmic dsRNA *(30)*.

The extraordinary efficiency and potency of RNAi, especially in worms and flies, suggests a catalytic nature of the interference reaction. Long periods of inhibition can be obtained by only a few trigger dsRNAs without shutting down the target gene transcription. The silencing persists through cell division and can spread to other untreated cells *(37,38)*. It even can be inherited by subsequent generations of worms *(39)*. The most likely mechanism that contributes this characteristic is the involvement of an RNA-dependent RNA polymerase (RdRP) in RNAi. This has been shown to be the case by two recent reports from Paterson and Fire groups *(40,41)*, in which these authors provided biochemical and genetic evidence that RdRP indeed plays an important role in the amplification of RNAi effect in *C. elegans*. An RdRP activity could amplify the trigger dsRNA by using the siRNAs as primers to convert mRNA into dsRNAs that are degraded to produce new siRNAs, termed secondary siRNAs. Because there is no clear homologous gene of RdRP in either the *Drosophila* or mammalian genomes, the involvement of RdRP in RNAi in higher eukaryotes remains speculative. The generation of secondary siRNAs can initiate "transitive" RNAi, in which sequences upstream of the original target complementary are degraded *(42)*. This phenomenon would reduce the specificity of RNAi and limit its application.

2. DSRNA ACTION IN THE NUCLEUS

Although dsRNA in the cytoplasm is generally thought to arise by virus infection, most naturally occurring antisense RNA is thought to occur within the nucleus *(43,44)*. This would be via either purposeful antisense regulation or by unintended transcriptional readthrough. Recent studies suggest that such nuclear antisense regulation might be far more prevalent in mammalian genomes that was heretofore realized. A systematic study of vertebrate mRNA sequences indicated that 2% or more of protein-encoding genes might be regulated by natural antisense transcripts *(45)*.

2.1. Nuclear Retention Induced by Hyper-Editing

So far there is no evidence that dsRNAs in the nucleus trigger the PKR, INF or 2', 5'-AS pathways, or RNA interference. Then what is the fate of dsRNA in this cellular compartment? Many claims have been made for the effects of nuclear antisense RNA, including transcriptional regulation, inhibition of splicing, and mRNA transport and induction of mRNA instability *(46)*. There have been reports that dsRNA-specific RNase *(47)* and RNA helicase activities *(48,49)* exist in the nucleus, but convincing evidence of a regulatory role of these enzymes in gene expression is still lacking.

The most likely fate of dsRNA induced by the formation of sense–antisense duplexes in the nucleus is to be acted on by a member of the class of enzymes known as adenosine deaminases that act on dsRNAs (ADARs) *(50)*. In eukaryotes, ADAR was first discovered in *Xenopus* oocytes as a dsRNA unwinding and modifying activity *(51,52)*. The enzyme was subsequently found to catalyze the conversion of adenosines to inosines *(53,54)* within dsRNA by the mechanism of hydrolytic deamination *(55)*, and to exist ubiquitously in all higher eukaryotic cells from *C. elegans* and *Drosophila* to mammalian cells *(56,57)*. dsRNA that has been edited by ADAR contains I-U basepairs, which destabilize the RNA duplex and may lead to partial or complete unwinding *(53)*.

Both deamination activity and the ADAR protein have been demonstrated to localize to the nucleus: cytoplasmic ADAR deamination activity has not been reported *(58)*. RNAi can be antagonized by A-to-I hyper-editing in vitro *(59)*,

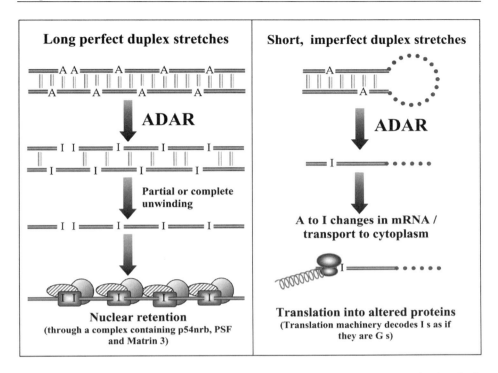

Fig. 3. ADAR effects depend on RNA structure and the length of the dsRNA duplex. Left: Promiscuous hyper-editing occurs on long duplex stretches. The two edited RNA strands are unwound and are retained within the nucleus. See text for details. Right: Short duplex stretches, mostly formed by a stem–loop structures, lead to specific editing, with only one or a few A to I changes. Such edited mRNAs can be transported to the cytoplasm, where they are translated into altered proteins.

further strengthening the hypothesis that RNAi does not act in the nucleus. ADAR editing of dsRNA is sensitive to the length of the duplex. Duplexes smaller than 15 bp are not edited in vitro, and optimal activity is seen with dsRNAs of 100 bp or longer (53,60,61). However, there are a number of reported editing substrates that lack long stretches of basepairing, illustrating that there are two modes of action of this enzyme, site-specific editing and promiscuous hyper-editing. Figure 3 illustrates the two types of editing carried out by ADAR.

Several cellular and viral mRNA targets which are specific edited by ADAR have been identified (62), including glutamate receptor, serotonin receptor, some *Drosophila* ion channel pre-mRNAs, and HDV antigenomic RNA (63–66). Specific editing alters one or a few As to Is, which leads to altered coding potential in mRNAs. One or a few amino acids in the protein encoded by specific edited mRNA will be changed, because Is are recognized as if they were Gs by the cellular translation machinery. Such a change can never create a translation stop codon, and so all A to I changes are missense in character. The editing generated amino acid alternation is usually critical for the normal function of the protein. The study using ADAR deletion mutants in *Drosophila* has suggested that specific A to I editing is primarily involved in nervous system function and integrity *(67)*. Mouse ADAR1 has been shown to be required for embryonic erythropoiesis *(68)*.

Long duplex RNA in nucleus can be promiscuously edited by ADAR, which causes about 50% of adenosines by modified to inosines with 5' neighbor base preference U>A>C>G *(69)*. A to I editing in the coding region of long dsRNA creates hypermutation, which, if translated, can generate mutant proteins, some of which might be hazardous to the cell *(1,70)*. Previous studies using the mouse polyoma virus system showed that hyper-edited viral RNA is specifically re-tained in the nucleus, in contrast to unedited RNA *(71)*. Thus, promiscuously edited RNA is not allowed to exit the nucleus. In polyoma virus-infected cells, natural antisense RNA to viral early transcripts is produced at late times in infection, accounting for a significant down regulation of early strand gene expression at late times in infection *(72,73)*. Extensive base modification of early messages was detected at late infection stage. Analysis of early strand sequences demonstrated that roughly half of the adenosines were altered to inosines or guanosines. Specific detection by different hybridization probes revealed that the hyper-edited messages are relatively stable, but accumulate within the nucleus. Could this cellular response to viral infection reflect a common mecha-nism to deal with dsRNA in all higher eukaryotic cells?

Recent studies using the *Xenopus* oocyte microinjection system suggest that this nuclear retention model may represent a general quality control mechanism for mRNA function in higher eukaryotic cells *(74)*. In this work a variety of edited and inosine-containing RNAs could not be exported from the nucleus to the cytoplasm. Splicing cannot overcome inosine-induced retention *(75,76)*. Further biochemical techniques were used to identify proteins from HeLa cell nuclear extracts that preferentially recognize inosine-containing RNAs (I-RNAs). There appears to be a single highly conserved and abundant nuclear protein, p54[nrb] *(77)*, which binds hyper-edited RNAs with a striking specificity *(74)*. This protein exists in a complex with the splicing factor PSF *(78,79)* and the inner nuclear matrix structural protein matrin 3 *(80,81)*, which confers highly cooperative binding to I-RNA and leads to nuclear retention, most likely via attachment to the nuclear matrix. p54[nrb] is the first identified nuclear RNA binding protein that requires inosine for high-affinity binding to RNA. This protein exists in a novel nuclear compartment *(82)* and has been shown to participate in multiple cellular activities, including transcription regulation *(83,84)* and pre-mRNA splicing *(77)*. Because of its unique substrate specific-ity, one important function of this protein appears to be to retain a specific subset of RNAs in the nucleus. These data have led to the important conclusion that nuclear antisense RNA leads to hyper-editing and subsequent nuclear retention of target transcripts.

2.2. Other Cellular Responses to dsRNA in Nucleus

The mechanism of many naturally nuclear antisense RNA in the regulation of gene expression has not been completely uncovered, such as the well-studied phenomenon–genomic imprinting *(85,86)* and X-chromosome inactivation, in which long nuclear antisense RNA has been suggested to play a critical role *(87)*. Genomic imprinting affects many mammalian genes and results in the expression of those genes from only one of the two parental chromosomes. So far, about 20% of known imprinted genes are associated with antisense transcripts, most of which are noncoding RNA and may have regulatory functions. A recent study from Sleutels et al. *(88)* showed that the *Air* antisense RNA overlapping the maternally expressed IGF2r has an active role and is required in genomic imprinting. So far there is no direct evidence for ADAR in genomic imprinting, but the detailed molecular mechanism of the function of antisense transcript is not yet understood.

A novel mechanism of gene silencing by dsRNA in the nucleus has been found in plant cells *(32,89,90)*, and involves *de novo* cytosine (C) methylation of homologous DNA sequences guided by dsRNA (RNA-directed DNA Methylation, or RdDM). This phenomenon was first discovered in viroid-infected transgenic plants and subsequently in nonpathogenic plant systems. This transcriptional gene silencing pathway shares some similarities with RNAi in animal cells, such that the dsRNAs are cleaved into siRNAs and only DNA sequences complementary to the guide RNA become modified *(91)*. An RNase-III-like enzyme, a *de novo* DNA methyltransferase, and an RNA helicase are believed to be involved in this process. DNA targets as short as 30 bp can be modified. DNA methylation can influence the binding of proteins to DNA, which in turn inhibits specific gene expression on transcription level. It has been suggested that the siRNA in RdDM could be generated in both the nucleus and the cytoplasm, presumably due to the absence of ADAR activity in plant cell nuclei. So far RdDM has not been detected in worms, flies, mice, or other animal cells, and there is little evidence that transcriptional gene silencing also exists in animals, though the possibility remains that this mechanism exists.

2.3. Natural Antisense RNAs That Might Act in the Nucleus

A large number of naturally occurring antisense transcripts have been reported in the literature (reviewed in ref. *1*), and several will be described briefly here. Basic fibroblast growth factor (bFGF) is a highly conserved and ubiquitously distributed mitogen. The bFGF gene locus is transcribed into several mRNA transcripts, including an antisense RNA derived from the opposite DNA strand.

This natural antisense RNA may function in the regulation of bFGF sense mRNA expression and turnover. The relative abundance of bFGF sense and antisense RNA varies in different tissues and different developmental stages, which suggests a regulatory role of this antisense strand in bFGF expression *(92–94)*.

The expression of *p53* also appears to be regulated at posttranscriptional level in some cells *(95)*. Khochbin and Lawrence *(96)* identified a 1.3kb polyadenylated nuclear RNA that span the first intron of the *p53* gene but in the antisense orientation, which likely inhibits the transport of the sense RNA to the cytoplasm.

Msx1 has been suggested to play a critical role in terminal cell differentiation and the development of tooth and craniofacial skeleton. Recently, an endogenous Msx1 antisense RNA in mice, rats, and humans has been identified *(97)*. In vivo studies showed that the balance between the levels of the two Msx1 sense–antisense RNAs is related to the expression of Msx1 protein, which suggests that the ratio between these two RNAs is a very important factor in the control of skeletal terminal differentiation. This antisense RNA appears to be polyadenylated, but the precise mechanism for Msx1 sense–antisense RNA physical interactions has not been defined. Both in vitro and in vivo data strongly suggest a down-regulation of Msx1 by the Msx1 antisense RNA.

Other antisense RNA regulation includes eIF-2α, *myc*, murine myelin basic protein and thyroid hormone receptor ErbAα/Rev-ErbAα et al. *(98–101)*. So far, however, the molecular mechanisms of action these antisense RNAs in the regulation of gene expression have not been uncovered *(102)*.

3. CONCLUSIONS

As we have seen, dsRNA has a variety of profound effects on cells, but these effects differ depending both on the intrinsic nature of the dsRNA trigger and on the cellular localization of the duplexes. Figure 4 presents our model for the various actions of dsRNA molecules in different cellular compartments, and summarized the major points stressed in this chapter. Characterization and understanding the different pathways of cellular responses to dsRNA will help in studies of not only the basic mechanism of dsRNA or antisense RNA in the regulation of cellular gene expression, but also in the design and implementation of effective antisense RNA strategies to inhibit target gene expression. When using antisense RNA as a tool to inhibit gene expression, many issues have to be addressed because of the complexities of cellular responses to dsRNAs as discussed here. Because long dsRNA in the cytoplasm triggers nonspecific inhibition of all gene expression owing to the PKR and IFN systems, and most designed antisense RNAs are relatively long, then for many mammalian cells, specifically silencing gene expression by antisense RNA should be targeted to the nucleus. One technology for doing this has been described *(72)*. In this method, antisense transcripts were retained in the nucleus by preventing their export (by inactivat-

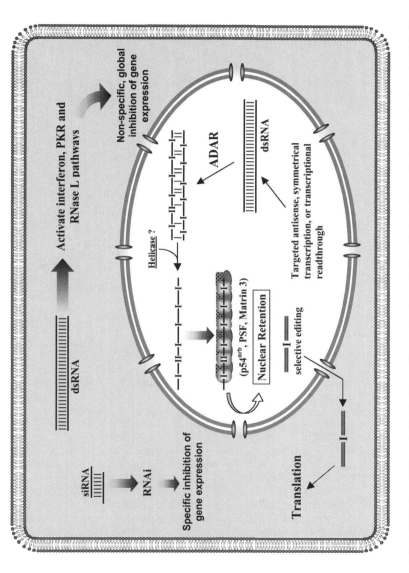

Fig. 4. Model: dsRNA has different effects depending not only on its length, but also on its location in the cell. This figure summarizes the major points made in the chapter, and these effects must be considered when designing effective antisense strategies.

ing 3'-end polyadenylation, which is important for mRNA export). If antisense RNA is expressed in the cytoplasm, then one must be aware of the consequences of its expression in this cellular compartment. If cytoplasmic localization in unavoidable, it would be wise to consider expressing very short duplexes, which would escape the very strong, and rather nonsequence-specific consequences of long cytoplasmic dsRNA.

ACKNOWLEDGMENTS

This work was supported by grant CA32325 from the National Cancer Institute to Gordon G. Carmichael.

REFERENCES

1. Kumar M, Carmichael GG. Antisense RNA: function and fate of duplex RNA in cells of higher eukaryotes. Microbiol Mol Biol Rev 1998; 62:1415–1434.
2. Bernstein E, Denli AM, Hannon GJ. The rest is silence. RNA 2001; 7:1509–1521.
3. Hammond SM, Caudy AA, Hannon GJ. Post-transcriptional gene silencing by double-stranded RNA. Nat Rev Genet 2001; 2:110–119.
4. Zamore PD. RNA interference: listening to the sound of silence. Nat Struct Biol 2001; 8:746–750.
5. Bass BL. Double-stranded RNA as a template for gene silencing. Cell 2000; 101:235–238.
6. Sharp PA. RNA interference—2001. Genes Dev 2001; 15:485–490.
7. Sen GC. Viruses and interferons. Annu Rev Microbiol 2001; 55:255–281.
8. Kalvakolanu DVR, Borden EC. An overview of the interferon system: signal transduction and mechanisms of action. Cancer Investig 1996; 14:25–53.
9. Pellegrini S, Schindler C. Early events in signalling by interferons. Trends Biochem Sci 1993; 18:338–342.
10. Proud CG. PKR: a new name and new roles. Trends Biochem Sci 1995; 20:241–246.
11. Robertson HD, Mathews MB. The regulation of the protein kinase PKR by RNA. Biochimie 1996; 78:909–914
12. Williams BR. Role of the double-stranded RNA-activated protein kinase (PKR) in cell regulation. Biochem Soc Trans 1997; 25:509–513.
13. Samuel CE, Kuhen KL, George CX, Ortega LG, Rende-Fournier R, Tanaka H. The PKR protein kinase—an interferon-inducible regulator of cell growth and differentiation. Int J Hematol 1997; 65:227–237.
14. Nanduri S, Carpick BW, Yang Y, Williams BR, Qin J. Structure of the double-stranded RNA-binding domain of the protein kinase PKR reveals the molecular basis of its dsRNA-mediated activation. EMBO J 1998; 17:5458–5465.
15. Nanduri S, Rahman F, Williams BR, Qin J. A dynamically tuned double-stranded RNA binding mechanism for the activation of antiviral kinase PKR. EMBO J 2000; 19:5567–5574.
16. Ung TL, Cao C, Lu J, Ozato K, Dever TE. Heterologous dimerization domains functionally substitute for the double-stranded RNA binding domains of the kinase PKR. EMBO J 2001; 20:3728–3737.
17. Kumar A, Haque J, Lacoste J, Hiscott J, Williams BR. Double-stranded RNA-dependent protein kinase activates transcription factor NF-kappa B by phosphorylating I kappa B. Proc Natl Acad Sci USA 1994; 91:6288–6292.
18. Samuel CE. Mechanism of interferon action: phosphorylation of protein synthesis initiation factor eIF-2 in interferon-treated human cells by a ribosome- associated kinase processing site

specificity similar to hemin-regulated rabbit reticulocyte kinase. Proc Natl Acad Sci USA 1979; 76:600–604.

19. Samuel CE. The eIF-2-alpha protein kinases, regulators of translation in eukaryotes from yeasts to humans. J Biol Chem 1993; 268:7603–7606.

20. Kerr IM, Brown RE. pppA2'p5'A2'p5'A: an inhibitor of protein synthesis synthesized with an enzyme fraction from interferon-treated cells. Proc Natl Acad Sci USA 1978; 75:256–260.

21. Baglioni C, Maroney PA, West DK. 2'5'Oligo(A) polymerase activity and inhibition of viral RNA synthesis in interferon-treated HeLa cells. Biochemistry 1979; 18:1765–1770.

22. Bisbal C, Salehzada T, Lebleu B, Bayard B. Characterization of two murine (2'-5')(A)n-dependent endonucleases of different molecular mass. Eur J Biochem 1989; 179:595–602.

23. Floyd-Smith G, Slattery E, Lengyel P. Interferon action: RNA cleavage pattern of a (2'-5') oligoadenylate-dependent endonuclease. Science 1981; 212:1030–1032.

24. Castelli JC, Hassel BA, Wood KA, et al. A study of the interferon antiviral mechanism: apoptosis activation by the 2-5A system. J Exp Med 1997; 186:967–972.

25. Zhou A, Paranjape J, Brown TL, et al. Interferon action and apoptosis are defective in mice devoid of 2',5'-oligoadenylate-dependent RNase L. EMBO J 1997; 16:6355–6363.

26. Fire A, Xu S, Montgomery MK, Kostas SA, Driver SE, Mello CC. Potent and specific genetic interference by double-stranded RNA in Caenorhabditis elegans. Nature 1998; 391:806–811.

27. Zamore PD, Tuschl T, Sharp PA, Bartel DP. RNAi: double-stranded RNA directs the ATP-dependent cleavage of mRNA at 21 to 23 nucleotide intervals. Cell 2000; 101:25–33.

28. Tuschl T, Zamore PD, Lehmann R, DP, Sharp PA. Targeted mRNA degradation by double-stranded RNA in vitro. Genes Dev 1999; 13:3191–3197.

29. Elbashir SM, Harborth J, Lendeckel W, Yalcin A, Weber K, Tuschl T. Duplexes of 21-nucleotide RNAs mediate RNA interference in cultured mammalian cells. Nature 2001; 411:494–498.

30. Paddison PJ, Caudy AA, Hannon GJ. Stable suppression of gene expression by RNAi in mammalian cells. Proc Natl Acad Sci USA 2002; 99:1443–1448.

31. Hammond SM, Bernstein E, Beach D, Hannon GJ. An RNA-directed nuclease mediates post-transcriptional gene silencing in Drosophila cells. Nature 2000; 404:293–296.

32. Matzke MA, Matzke AJ, Pruss GJ, Vance VB. RNA-based silencing strategies in plants. Curr Opin Genet Dev 2001; 11:221–227.

33. Bernstein E, Caudy AA, Hammond SM, Hannon GJ. Role for a bidentate ribonuclease in the initiation step of RNA interference. Nature 2001; 409:363–366.

34. Nykanen A, Haley B, Zamore PD. ATP requirements and small interfering RNA structure in the RNA interference pathway. Cell 2001; 107:309–321.

35. Billy E, Brondani V, Zhang H, Muller U, Filipowicz W. Specific interference with gene expression induced by long, double-stranded RNA in mouse embryonal teratocarcinoma cell lines. Proc Natl Acad Sci USA 2001; 98:14428–14433.

36. Bitko V, Barik S. Phenotypic silencing of cytoplasmic genes using sequence-specific double-stranded short interfering RNA and its application in the reverse genetics of wild type negative-strand RNA viruses. BMC Microbiol 2001; 1:34.

37. Tabara H, Sarkissian M, Kelly WG, et al. The rde-1 gene, RNA interference, and transposon silencing in C. elegans. Cell 1999; 99:123–132.

38. Tabara H, Grishok A, Mello CC. RNAi in C. elegans: soaking in the genome sequence. Science 1998; 282:430–431.

39. Grishok A, Tabara H, Mello CC. Genetic requirements for inheritance of RNAi in C. elegans. Science 2000; 287:2494–2497.

40. Lipardi C, Wei Q, Paterson BM. RNAi as random degradative PCR: siRNA primers convert mRNA into dsRNAs that are degraded to generate new siRNAs. Cell 2001; 107:297–307.

41. Sijen T, Fleenor J, Simmer F, et al. On the role of RNA amplification in dsRNA-triggered gene silencing. Cell 2001; 107:465–476.

42. Nishikura K. A short primer on RNAi: RNA-directed RNA polymerase acts as a key catalyst. Cell 2001; 107:415–418.
43. Cornelissen M. Nuclear and cytoplasmic sites for anti-sense control. Nucleic Acids Res 1989; 17:7203–7209.
44. Murray JAH, Crockett N. Antisense techniques: an overview. In: Murray JAH, ed. Modern Cell Biology. New York: Wiley-Liss, 1992:1–49.
45. Lehner B, Williams G, Campbell RD, Sanderson CM. Antisense transcripts in the human genome. Trends Genet 2002; 18:63–65.
46. Denhardt DT. Mechanism of action of antisense RNA. Sometime inhibition of transcription, processing, transport, or translation. Ann NY Acad Sci 1992; 660:70–76.
47. Wu H, MacLeod AR, Lima WF, Crooke ST. Identification and partial purification of human double strand RNase activity. A novel terminating mechanism for oligoribonucleotide antisense drugs. J Biol Chem 1998; 273:2532–2542.
48. Staley JP, Guthrie C. Mechanical devices of the spliceosome: motors, clocks, springs, and things. Cell 1998; 92:315–326.
49. Wassarman DA, Steitz JA. RNA splicing—alive with DEAD proteins. Nature 1991; 349:463–464.
50. Bass BL, Nishikura K, Keller W, et al. A standardized nomenclature for adenosine deaminases that act on RNA. RNA 1997; 3:947–949.
51. Bass BL, Weintraub H. A developmentally regulated activity that unwinds RNA duplexes. Cell 1987; 48:607–613.
52. Rebagliati MR, Melton DA. Antisense RNA injections in fertilized frog eggs reveal an RNA duplex unwinding activity. Cell 1987; 48:599–605.
53. Bass BL, Weintraub H. An unwinding activity that covalently modifies its double-stranded RNA substrate. Cell 1988; 55:1089–1098.
54. Wagner RW, Smith JE, Cooperman BS, Nishikura K. A double-stranded RNA unwinding activity introduces structural alterations by means of adenosine to inosine conversions in mammalian cells and Xenopus eggs. Proc Natl Acad Sci USA 1989; 86:2647–2651.
55. Polson AG, Crain PF, Pomerantz SC, McCloskey JA, Bass BL. The mechanism of adenosine to inosine conversion by the double-stranded RNA unwinding/modifying activity: a high-performance liquid chromatography-mass spectrometry analysis. Biochemistry 1991; 30:11507–11514.
56. Morse DP, Bass BL. Long RNA hairpins that contain inosine are present in Caenorhabditis elegans poly(A)+ RNA. Proc Natl Acad Sci USA 1999; 96:6048–6053.
57. Wagner RW, Yoo C, Wrabetz L, et al. Double-stranded RNA unwinding and modifying activity is detected ubiquitously in primary tissues and cell lines. Mol Cell Biol 1990; 10:5586–5590.
58. Saccomanno L, Bass BL. The cytoplasm of Xenopus oocytes contains a factor that protects double-stranded RNA from adenosine-to-inosine modification. Mol Cell Biol 1994; 14:5425–5432.
59. Scadden AD, Smith CW. RNAi is antagonized by A-to-I hyper-editing. EMBO Rep 2001; 2:1107–1111.
60. Nishikura K. Modulation of double-stranded RNAs in vivo by RNA duplex unwindase. Ann NY Acad Sci 1992; 660:240–250.
61. Lehmann KA, Bass BL. The importance of internal loops within RNA substrates of ADAR1. J Mol Biol 1999; 291:1–13.
62. Keegan LP, Gallo A, O'Connell MA. The many roles of an RNA editor. Nat Rev Genet 2001; 2:869–878.
63. Sommer B, Kohler M, Sprengel R, Seeburg PH. RNA editing in brain controls a determinant of ion flow in glutamate-gated channels. Cell 1991; 67:11–19.

64. Burns CM, Chu H, Rueter SM, et al. Regulation of serotonin-2C receptor G-protein coupling by RNA editing. Nature 1997; 387:303–308.

65. Polson AG, Bass BL, Casey JL. RNA editing of hepatitis delta virus antigenome by dsRNA-adenosine deaminase. Nature 1996; 380:454–456.

66. Wong SK, Sato S, Lazinski DW. Substrate recognition by ADAR1 and ADAR2. RNA 2001; 7:846–858.

67. Palladino MJ, Keegan LP, O'Connell MA, Reenan RA. A-to-I pre-mRNA editing in Drosophila is primarily involved in adult nervous system function and integrity. Cell 2000; 102:437–449.

68. Wang Q, Khillan J, Gadue P, Nishikura K. Requirement of the RNA editing deaminase ADAR1 gene for embryonic erythropoiesis. Science 2000; 290:1765–1768.

69. Polson AG, Bass BL. Preferential selection of adenosines for modification by double-stranded RNA adenosine deaminase. EMBO J 1994; 13:5701–5711.

70. Bass BL. RNA editing and hypermutation by adenosine deamination. Trends Biochem Sci 1997; 22:157–162.

71. Kumar M, Carmichael GG. Nuclear antisense RNA induces extensive adenosine modifications and nuclear retention of target transcripts. Proc Natl Acad Sci USA 1997; 94:3542–3547.

72. Liu Z, Batt DB, Carmichael GG. Targeted nuclear antisense RNA mimics natural antisense-induced degradation of polyoma virus early RNA. Proc Natl Acad Sci USA 1994; 91:4258–4262.

73. Liu Z, Carmichael GG. Nuclear antisense RNA: An efficient new method to inhibit gene expression. Mol Biotechnol 1994; 2:107–118.

74. Zhang Z, Carmichael GG. The fate of dsRNA in the nucleus. A p54(nrb)-containing complex mediates the nuclear retention of promiscuously A-to-I edited RNAs. Cell 2001; 106:465–475.

75. Zhou Z, Luo M, Straesser K, Katahira J, Hurt E, Reed R. The protein Aly links pre-messenger-RNA splicing to nuclear export in metazoans. Nature 2000; 407:401–405.

76. Luo M, Reed R. Splicing is required for rapid and efficient mRNA export in Metazoans. PNAS 1999; 96:14937–14942.

77. Dong B, Horowitz DS, Kobayashi R, Krainer AR. Purification and cDNA cloning of HeLa cell p54nrb, a nuclear protein with two RNA recognition motifs and extensive homology to human splicing factor PSF and Drosophila NONA/BJ6. Nucleic Acids Res 1993; 21:4085–4092.

78. Gozani O, Patton JG, Reed R. A novel set of spliceosome-associated proteins and the essential splicing factor PSF bind stably to pre-mRNA prior to catalytic step II of the splicing reaction. EMBO J 1994; 13:3356–3367.

79. Patton JG, Porro EB, Galceran J, Tempst P, Nadal-Ginard B. Cloning and characterization of PSF, a novel pre-mRNA splicing factor. Genes Dev 1993; 7:393–406.

80. Belgrader P, Dey R, Berezney R. Molecular cloning of matrin 3. A 125-kilodalton protein of the nuclear matrix contains an extensive acidic domain. J Biol Chem 1991; 266:9893–9899.

81. Nakayasu H, Berezney R. Nuclear matrins: identification of the major nuclear matrix proteins. Proc Natl Acad Sci USA 1991; 88:10312–10316.

82. Fox AH, Lam YW, Leung AK, et al. Paraspeckles. A novel nuclear domain. Curr Biol 2002; 12:13–25.

83. Yang YS, Hanke JH, Carayannopoulos L, Craft CM, Capra JD, Tucker PW. NonO, a non-POU-domain-containing, octamer-binding protein, is the mammalian homolog of Drosophila nonAdiss. Mol Cell Biol 1993; 13:5593–5603.

84. Yang YS, Yang MC, Tucker PW, Capra JD. NonO enhances the association of many DNA-binding proteins to their targets. Nucleic Acids Res 1997; 25:2284–2292.

85. Tilghman SM. The sins of the fathers and mothers: genomic imprinting in mammalian development. Cell 1999; 96:185–193.

86. Reik W, Walter J. Genomic imprinting: parental influence on the genome. Nat Rev Genet 2001; 2:21–32.
87. Mlynarczyk SK, Panning B. X inactivation: Tsix and Xist as yin and yang. Curr Biol 2000; 10:R899–903.
88. Sleutels F, Zwart R, Barlow DP. The non-coding Air RNA is required for silencing autosomal imprinted genes. Nature 2002; 415:810–813.
89. Vance V, Vaucheret H. RNA silencing in plants—defense and counterdefense. Science 2001; 292:2277–2280.
90. Vaucheret H, Fagard M. Transcriptional gene silencing in plants: targets, inducers and regulators. Trends Genet 2001; 17:29–35.
91. Mette MF, Aufsatz W, van Der Winden J, Matzke MA, Matzke AJ. Transcriptional silencing and promoter methylation triggered by double-stranded RNA. EMBO J 2000; 19:5194–5201.
92. Volk R, Koster M, Poting A, Hartmann L, Knochel W. An antisense transcript from the Xenopus laevis bFGF gene coding for an evolutionarily conserved 24 kd protein. EMBO J 1989; 8:2983–2988.
93. Murphy PR, Knee RS. Identification and characterization of an antisense RNA transcript (gfg) from the human basic fibroblast growth factor gene. Mol Endocrinol 1994; 8:852–859.
94. Knee RS, Pitcher SE, Murphy PR. Basic fibroblast growth factor sense (FGF) and antisense (gfg) RNA transcripts are expressed in unfertilized human oocytes and in differentiated adult tissues. Biochem Biophys Res Commun 1994; 205:577–583.
95. Dony C, Kessel M, Gruss P. Post-transcriptional control of myc and p53 expression during differentiation of the embryonal carcinoma cell line F9. Nature 1985; 317:636–639.
96. Khochbin S, Lawrence JJ. An antisense RNA involved in p53 mRNA maturation in murine erythroleukemia cells induced to differentiate. EMBO J 1989; 8:4107–4114.
97. Blin-Wakkach C, Lezot F, Ghoul-Mazgar S, et al. Endogenous Msx1 antisense transcript: in vivo and in vitro evidences, structure, and potential involvement in skeleton development in mammals. Proc Natl Acad Sci USA 2001; 98:7336–7341.
98. Silverman TA, Noguchi M, Safer B. Role of sequences within the first intron in the regulation of expression of eukaryotic initiation factor 2 alpha. J Biol Chem 1992; 267:9738–9742.
99. Krystal GW, Armstrong BC, Battey JF. N-myc mRNA forms an RNA-RNA duplex with endogenous antisense transcripts. Mol Cell Biol 1990; 10:4180–4191.
100. Okano H, Ikenaka K, Mikoshiba K. Recombination within the upstream gene of duplicated myelin basic protein genes of myelin deficient shimld mouse results in the production of antisense RNA. EMBO J 1988; 7:3407–3412.
101. Lazar MA, Hodin RA, Darling DS, Chin WW. A novel member of the thyroid/steroid hormone receptor family is encoded by the opposite strand of the rat c-erbA alpha transcriptional unit. Mol Cell Biol 1989; 9:1128–1136.
102. Knee R, Murphy PR. Regulation of gene expression by natural antisense RNA transcripts. Neurochem Int 1997; 31:379–392.

III DELIVERY

8 The Transport of Oligonucleotides Into Cells

R. L. Juliano, PhD

CONTENTS

1. INTRODUCTION

This is a critical and exciting period in the development of antisense oligo-nucleotides (ONs) as therapeutic agents. Recently, there has been substantial progress in developing newer, more effective chemistries for ONs *(1)*. Ongoing clinical trials using antisense have yielded promising results, particularly in the context of cancer therapy *(2)*. Finally, important new roles for antisense as a tool in drug discovery have emerged *(3)*. However, continued progress in antisense therapeutics and drug discovery remains contingent on a fuller understanding of the processes that control the entry of ONs into cells and tissues. Because the target sites for antisense drugs are in the nucleus and cytoplasm, efficient transport of ONs into these compartments is a key aspect of effective therapy. In this chapter, I will examine some of the basic information concerning the cellular uptake and transport of ONs and briefly discuss some strategies for enhancing delivery of antisense compounds into cells. Other recent reviews have also dealt with these issues *(4,5)*.

From: *Cancer Drug Discovery and Development:*
Nucleic Acid Therapeutics in Cancer
Edited by: A. M. Gewirtz © Humana Press Inc., Totowa, NJ

2. BASIC ASPECTS OF ON TRANSPORT

From the point of view of basic membrane biochemistry, it is actually quite remarkable that antisense compounds work at all. Cell membranes are intended by nature to be very impermeable to large, polar molecules such as ONs, unless specific transporter systems are involved. When administered as "free" molecules (in the absence of any delivery agent), most types of ONs are initially accumulated in cells due to one form or another of endocytosis (6,7). Use of fluorescent labeling has indicated that ONs are localized in cytoplasmic endosomes, and little fluorescence is associated with the nucleus at early time points. By contrast, when fluorescent ONs are directly micro-injected into the cytoplasm, they rapidly enter the nucleus (8). This suggests that release from endosomes may be a rate-limiting step for antisense effects in most cell types. Although many cells take up ONs by endocytotic mechanisms, there is quite a variation between cell types. For example, in polarized epithelial cells differences in uptake in the apical and basolateral regions have been noted (9), whereas unusually high uptake rates have been seen in keratinocytes (10).

3. INTERACTIONS OF ONS WITH MEMBRANES

The basic mechanism of entry low-molecular-weight drugs into the cell is diffusion across the lipid bilayer of the plasma membrane. However, in the case of typical anionic ONs, it is unlikely that these highly charged molecules can directly diffuse through the hydrophobic bilayer. There are a number of chemically modified ONs that are uncharged; for example, methyphosphonates, peptide-nucleic acids (PNAs), and morpholino compounds (11). There are also ONs with nonpolar substituents, including cholesterol and alkyl chains, intended to increase membrane binding and permeation. Although it is conceivable that such uncharged or modified ONs might readily enter cells by passive diffusion across the lipid bilayer, experience thus far suggests otherwise. For example, using liposomes as a model membrane system, it was found that both charged ONs and uncharged methylphosphonate compounds exhibited extremely slow diffusion rates across the lipid bilayer membrane (12). Other studies using alkyl-substituted ONs or uncharged PNAs also failed to demonstrate rapid passage across the lipid bilayer (13). Thus, even for uncharged ON derivatives, permeation by simple diffusion across the lipid bilayer is very slow. Against this, recent observations have demonstrated greater intracellular effects of "free" uncharged morpholino and PNA ONs, as compared to equally stable "free" anionic 2'-alkyl modified ONs (14,15). However, relatively high concentrations of ONs were used, and the onset of biological action was slow. Thus, there is probably some gradual penetration of uncharged ONs across membranes and into cytoplasmic and nuclear compartments. However, it is unclear if the transport is across the plasma membrane or whether it is composed of leaks from endosomal vesicles.

4. MEMBRANE RECEPTORS FOR ONS

The binding of ONs to cell-surface receptors would tend to enhance ON entry into cells in two ways. First, it would simply increase the local concentration of ON at the cell membrane. Second, if the receptor were linked to an active internalization pathway, this process would deliver the ON to the cell interior (although it still might be enclosed in a membrane-bound compartment).

Cell-surface proteins that bind ONs were first detected more than a decade ago and were described as molecules in the 80 kD range; these putative receptors were never well characterized (reviewed in ref. *16*). More recently, a variety of potential ON binding proteins ranging from 40 to 60 kD have been detected, but most of these also remain poorly characterized *(6,17,18)*. Proteins with a high binding affinity for polyanionic molecules are likely candidates as cellular receptors for ONs. Thus, MAC-1 (CD11b/CD18), a member of the β2 integrin subfamily that is known to bind avidly to heparin-like molecules, has emerged as an interesting ON receptor *(19)*. Another interesting finding was the identification of so-called scavenger receptors (also known to bind polyanions) as being potentially important ON receptors, especially in the liver and kidney *(20,21)*. However, studies using mice genetically defective in one form of scavenger receptor have suggested that this receptor plays only a minor role in determining the overall clearance and tissue distribution of ONs in vivo *(22)*. Another very intriguing finding concerns interactions of bacterial DNA with *Toll*-like receptors on mammalian cells *(23)*. These receptors are clearly involved in the immune-stimulatory actions of prokaryotic dsDNA; however, the role of this receptor class in uptake of ss-ONs is not yet clearly defined. Several years ago there was a description of a protein(s) claimed as an actual transporter for ONs *(24)*. This description was based on the reconstitution of the protein into model planar lipid bilayers, so that electrophysiological measurements could be made. Incorporation of the binding protein into the bilayer resulted in ion channel activity where the current was carried by the ON. Recently, the same group has made additional progress in identifying the elements of the transporter system *(25)*. This interesting set of observations raises a number of questions, including whether the transporter, while being detectable by sensitive biophysical measurements, actually plays a significant role in ON uptake into cells.

In addition to uptake by endogenous ON receptors, investigators have coupled ONs to peptides designed to bind to specific cell-surface receptors, thus promoting uptake of the ON complex. For example, peptides designed to bind to integrins *(26)* or to insulin-like growth factor-1 receptor *(27)* have been used to enhance ON uptake. In summary, a variety of potential cell-surface receptors for ONs have been identified, as well as possible transporters. Despite the variety of potential binding proteins, receptors, and transporters, it should be noted, that careful studies of ON uptake by cells continues to confirm the basic observation that most uptake occurs via endocytotic pathways, although these may differ somewhat from classical routes of endocytosis *(28)*.

5. METHODS FOR ENHANCING THE INTRACELLULAR DELIVERY OF ONS

There is an interesting dichotomy between studies of antisense in cultured cells and those in animals and patients. For the most part, in vivo studies have used free ONs, whereas cell-culture studies have required some sort of delivery agent for effective action. Although a number of possible spurious results may have occurred in some in vivo studies, it is also clear that genuine antisense actions have been attained in this context. The reasons for this dichotomy are unclear. One possibility is that the more protracted in vivo studies allow gradual accumulation of intracellular pools of ONs that eventual leak from membrane-bound compartments to the cytoplasm and nucleus. Thus, it is not clear that one needs to use delivery approaches in antisense therapeutics. On the other hand, thus far there have not been thorough studies of whether the current rather modest therapeutic effects attained by antisense could be further enhanced using delivery modalities. Therefore, it seems worthwhile to consider ON delivery strategies for potential therapeutic applications.

5.1. Cationic Lipids, Nanoparticles, and Dendrimers

One of the most popular strategies for enhancing the delivery of ONs to cells is the use of various particulate or polymeric delivery agents. Thus, cationic lipids have been the "gold standard" for delivery of ONs (including both antisense and siRNA), and new forms are constantly being developed *(29)*. Despite their utility in cell culture, cationic lipids present a number of problems for in vivo utilization including toxicity and a tendency to be rapidly cleared by the phagocytes of the reticuloendothelial system rather than being able to enter a variety of tissues. Several types of polymeric nanoparticles with embedded or absorbed ONs have also been studied *(30)*; however, some of the same issues apply to these systems as to the cationic lipid systems. Polycationic dendrimers have also been examined as a potential delivery modality *(5,31)*. The dendrimer–ON complexes seem to be somewhat less effective in cell culture than cationic lipid complexes; however, they offer the advantage of being smaller in size and thus more likely to traverse the circulation and enter tissues. Indeed, dendrimers are being examined for in vivo use as radiographic contrast agents *(32)*, suggesting an ability to attain excellent tissue penetration.

5.2. Low-Molecular-Weight Delivery Systems

In addition to the macromolecular and supramolecular complexes mentioned above, there have also been several examples of enhancing ON delivery using reagents of relatively low-molecular mass. For example, complexation with cyclodextrins seems a straightforward and pragmatic approach *(33)*. However, the effects attained thus far have been relatively modest. Recently, a lot of excitement has been generated concerning the use of various cell-penetrating or membrane-transducing peptides that have the ability to penetrate cell membranes and to bring along covalently attached peptides, ONs, and even proteins. This exciting area has been the subject of several recent reviews *(34,35)*. Importantly, in the context of this chapter, the use of conjugates of cell-penetrating peptides with ONs has led to some impressive results with both PNAs and with phosphorothioate antisense ONs *(36–38)*. A disadvantage with this approach is that the synthesis and purification of peptide–ON conjugates is complicated and expensive.

5.3. Sustained Release

An area of antisense pharmacology that is just beginning to be developed concerns the use of various polymeric sustained-release formulations. This topic has been dealt with in some recent reviews *(39,40)*. This is a promising avenue to explore because it could address issues such as the uptake of ONs from the gastrointestinal tract and the delivery of ONs by the transdermal route.

In summary, a variety of approaches are being developed to enhance the cellular and tissue delivery of ONs. When coupled with the latest advances in ON chemistry, these approaches could make important contributions to antisense therapeutics.

REFERENCES

1. Manoharan M. Oligonucleotide conjugates as potential antisense drugs with improved uptake, biodistribution, targeted delivery, and mechanism of action. Antisense Nucleic Acid Drug Dev 2002; 12:103–128.
2. Flahery KT, Stevenson JP, O'Dwyer PJ. Antisense therapeutics: lessons from early clinical trials. Curr Opin in Oncology 2001; 13:499–505
3. Dean NM. Functional genomics and target validation approaches using antisense oligonucleotide technology. Curr Opin in Biotechnology 2001; 12:622–625
4. Bennett CF. Antisense oligonucleotides: is the glass half full or half empty? Biochem Pharmacol 1998; 55:9–19.
5. Juliano RL, Alahari S, Yoo H, Kole R, Cho M. Antisense pharmacodynamics: critical issues in the transport and delivery of antisense oligonucleotides. Pharm Res 1999; 16:494–501
6. Beltinger C, Saragovi HU, Smith RM, et al. Binding, uptake and intracellular trafficking of phosphorothioate-modified oligodeoxynucleotides. J Clin Invest 1995; 95:1814–1823.
7. Shoji Y, Akhtar S, Periasamy A, Herman B, Juliano RL. Mechanism of cellular uptake of modified oligodeoxynucleotides containing methylphosphonate linkages. Nucleic Acids Research 1991; 19:5543–5550.
8. Leonetti JP, Mechti N, Degols G, Gagnor C, LeBleu B. Intracellular distribution of microinjected antisense oligonucleotides. Proc Natl Acad Sci USA 1991; 88:2702–2706.
9. Takakura Y, Oka Y, Hashida M. Cellular uptake properties of oligonucleotides in LLC-PK1 renal epithelial cells. Antisense Nucleic Acid Drug Dev 1998; 8:67–73.

10. Laktionov PP, Dazard JE, Vives E, et al. Characterisation of membrane oligonucleotide-binding proteins and oligonucleotide uptake in keratinocytes. Nucleic Acids Res 1999; 27:2315–2324

11. Matteucci M. Structural modifications toward improved antisense oligonucleotides. Drug Discovery and Design 1996; 4:1–16.

12. Akhtar S, Juliano RL. Permeation characteristics of antisense DNA oligonucleotide analogs across model membranes (Liposomes). Nucleic Acids Res 1991; 19:5551–5559.

13. Hughes JA, Bennett CF, Cook PD, Guinosso CJ, Mirabelli CK, Juliano RL. Lipid membrane permeability of 2'-modified derivatives of phosphorothioate oligonucleotides. J Pharm Sci 1994; 83:597–600.

14. Schmajuk G, Sierakowska H, Kole R. Antisense oligonucleotides with different back-bones. Modification of splicing pathways and efficacy of uptake. J Biol Chem 1999; 274:21783–21789.

15. Sazani P, Kang SH, Maier MA, et al. Nuclear antisense effects of neutral, anionic and cationic oligonucleotide analogs. Nucleic Acids Res 2001, 29:3965–3974.

16. Akhtar S, Juliano RL. Cellular uptake and intracellular fate of antisense oligonucleotides. Trends Cell Biol 1992; 2:139–143.

17. Laktionov PP, Dazard JE, Vives E, et al. Characterisation of membrane oligonucleotide-binding proteins and oligonucleotide uptake in keratinocytes. Nucleic Acids Res 1999; 27:2315–2324.

18. Corrias S, Cheng YC. Interaction of human plasma membrane proteins and oligodeoxy-nucleotides. Biochem Pharmacol 1998; 55:1221–1227.

19. Benimetskaya L, Loike JD, Khaled Z, et al. Mac-1 (CD11b/CD18) is an oligodeoxynucleotide-binding protein. Nat Med 1997; 3:414–420.

20. Biessen EA, Vietsch H, Kuiper J, Bijsterbosch MK, Berkel TJ. Liver uptake of phosphodiester oligodeoxynucleotides is mediated by scavenger receptors. Mol. Pharmacol. 1998, 53:262–269.

21. Steward A, Christian RA, Hamilton KO, Nicklin PL. Co-administration of polyanions with a phosphorothioate oligonucleotide (CGP 69846A): a role for the scavenger receptor in its in vivo disposition. Biochem Pharmacol 1998; 56:509–516.

22. Butler M, Crooke RM, Graham MJ, et al. Phosphorothioate oligodeoxynucleotides distribute similarly in class A scavenger receptor knockout and wild-type mice. J Pharmacol Exp Ther 2000; 292:489–496.

23. Hemmi H, Takeuchi O, Kawai T, et al. A Toll-like receptor recognizes bacterial DNA. Nature 2000; 408:740–745.

24. Hanss B, Leal-Pinto E, Bruggeman LA, Copeland TD, Klotman PE. Identification and characterization of a cell membrane nucleic acid channel. Proc Natl Acad Sci USA 1998; 95:1921–1926.

25. Hanss B, Leal-Pinto E, Teixeira A, et al. Cytosolic malate dehydrogenase confers selectivity of the nucleic acid-conducting channel. Proc Natl Acad Sci USA 2002; 99:1707–1712.

26. Bachmann AS, Surovoy A, Jung G, Moelling K. Integrin receptor-targeted transfer peptides for efficient delivery of antisense oligodeoxynucleotides. J Mol Med 1998; 76:126–132.

27. Basu S, Wickstrom E. Synthesis and characterization of a peptide nucleic acid conjugated to a D-peptide analog of insulin-like growth factor 1 for increased cellular uptake. Bioconjug Chem 1997; 8:481–488.

28. de Diesbach P, N'Kuli F, Berens C, et al. Receptor-mediated endocytosis of phosphodiester oligonucleotides in the HepG2 cell line: evidence for non-conventional intracellular trafficking Nucleic Acids Res 2002; 30:1512–1521.

29. Bennett CF, Mirejovsky D, Crooke RM, et al. Structural requirements for cationic lipid mediated phosphorothioate oligonucleotides delivery to cells in culture. J Drug Target 1998; 5:149–162.

30. Lambert G, Fattal E, Couvreur P. Nanoparticulate systems for the delivery of antisense oligonucleotides. Adv Drug Deliv Rev 2001; 47:99–112

31. Yoo H, Sazani P, Juliano RL. PAMAM dendrimers as delivery agents for antisense oligonucleotides. Pharm Res 1999; 16:1799–1804

32. Sato N, Kobayashi H, Hiraga A., et al. Pharmacokinetics and enhancement patterns of macromolecular MR contrast reagents with various sizes of polyamidoamine dendrimer cores. Mag Reson in Med 2001; 46:1169–1173

33. Redenti E, Pietra C, Gerloczy A, Szente L. Cyclodextrins in oligonucleotide delivery. Adv Drug Deliv Rev 2001; 53:235–244

34. Lindgren M, Hallbrink M, Prochiantz A, Langel U. Cell-penetrating peptides. Trends Pharm Sci 2000; 21:99–103.

35. Juliano RL, Astriab-Fisher A, Falke D. Macromolecular therapeutics: Emerging strategies for drug discovery in the postgenome era. Molecular Interventions 2002; 1:40–53

36. Pooga M, Soomets U, Hallbrink M, et al. Cell penetrating PNA constructs regulate galanin receptor levels and modify pain transmission in vivo. Nat Biotechnol 1998; 16:857–861.

37. Aldrian-Herrada G, Desarmenien MG, Orcel H, et al. A peptide nucleic acid (PNA) is more rapidly internalized in cultured neurons when coupled to a retro-inverso delivery peptide. The antisense activity depresses the target mRNA and protein in magnocellular oxytocin neurons. Nucleic Acids Res 1998; 26:4910–4916.

38. Astriab-Fisher A, Sergueev DS, Fisher M, Shaw BR, Juliano RL. Antisense inhibition of P-glycoprotein expression using peptide-oligonucleotide conjugates. Biochem Pharmacol 2000; 60:83–90.

39. Hughes MD, Hussain M, Nawaz Q, Sayyed P, Akhtar S. The cellular delivery of antisense oligonucleotides and ribozymes. Drug Discov Today 2001; 6:303–315.

40. Chirila TV, Rakoczy PE, Garrett KL, Lou X, Constable IJ. The use of synthetic polymers for delivery of therapeutic antisense oligodeoxynucleotides. Biomaterials 2002; 23:321–42.

9

Peptide-Mediated Delivery of Antisense Oligonucleotides and Related Material

Eric Vivès, PhD,
Jean Philippe Richard, MSc,
and Bernard Lebleu, PhD

1. INTRODUCTION

1.1. Nucleic Acids-Based Strategies to Control Gene Expression

Despite their simple conceptual basis, antisense strategies turned out more difficult to implement than initially anticipated. Overwhelming enthusiasm in academic laboratories and in the biotechnology industry in the early 1990s has been followed by a wave of skepticism about the real potential of nucleic acids-based drugs. An antisense oligonucleotide (ON)-based drug has been approved for the treatment of ocular cytomegalovirus infection, and several clinical trials are now well advanced for the treatment of various cancers and infectious diseases (as reviewed in ref. *1*). On the other hand, rapid progresses in genome and

From: *Cancer Drug Discovery and Development:*
Nucleic Acid Therapeutics in Cancer
Edited by: A. M. Gewirtz © Humana Press Inc., Totowa, NJ

transcriptome analysis have given a new impetus to the field when it was realized that the antisense approach might be a strategy of choice for functional genomics and for therapeutic target validation.

Although antisense strategies remain by far the most widely used, synthetic ONs (and their numerous analogs) allow control of gene expression in various ways. Triple-helix-forming ONs have been used to control transcription initiation (or elongation), or to induce site-specific mutations *(2)*. Double-stranded ON (or decoy ON) have been used in vitro and in vivo to titrate several transcription factors *(see* ref. *3* for a review).

The catalytic properties of some RNA motifs, and in particular of the hammerhead and hairpin ribozymes, have already led to several applications. Along the same lines, RNA-cleaving catalytic DNA motifs (or DNAzymes) with exquisite sequence specificity have recently been selected from combinatorial DNA libraries *(see* ref. *4* for a review).

Finally, double-stranded RNA-mediated silencing of gene expression (a phenomenon named RNA interference [RNAi]) has emerged as a promising tool to analyze gene function. Initially described in plants and in invertebrates (as *Drosophila* or *Caenorhabditis elegans*), RNAi has very recently been applied to mammalian cells as well, provided short (21 nt long) double-stranded RNAs (or siRNA) are used. Although the underlying mechanisms are still far to be understood, the dsRNA trigger appears to act as a guide to promote the specific degradation of homologous mRNA when siRNA are used. Gene-specific silencing is, on the contrary, buried in nonspecific responses (the interferon-triggered RNase L and PKR pathways) when longer dsRNA are used [5]).

1.2. Appropriate Delivery May Solve Problems Encountered in the Implementation of Antisense Strategies

Several unexpected problems have slowed down or complicated the implementation of antisense strategies. Most will probably be encountered in the use of other synthetic ON-based strategies as well. In a nutshell, major problems have been as follow:

1. The difficulty to select the most appropriate target site for an ON when dealing with the unknown three-dimensional structure of a mRNA.
2. The degradation of unprotected nucleic acids by nucleases in biological and cellular fluids.
3. The poor efficiency with which nucleic acids are taken up by most cell lines, although some primary cells might internalize ON more efficiently than cell lines.
4. The unexpected side effects linked with some motifs in antisense ON, as for instance the activation of antigen-presenting cells by CpG-containing ON (*see* ref. *6* for a review).

With the exception of the first one, these limitations could in theory be partly overcome by the association of synthetic ON with appropriate delivery vehicles. As an example, early studies with HIV-1-specific phosphorothioate antisense analogs turned out disappointing in cell culture models. Phosphoro-thioate ON derivatives indeed led to nonspecific effects (common to sulfated polyanions), which masked the sequence-specific antiviral activity, and phosphodiester ON were not effective since they were too rapidly degraded. Poly L-lysine conjugated phosphodiester ON did promote an antiviral response whose specificity was attested by the ability to discriminate sequence heterogeneity among two HIV-1 isolates *(7)*.

In addition, appropriate delivery should in principle be able to control more adequately the biodistribution of ON (*see* ref. *8* for a review). As an example, a phosphorothioate ON derivative was more efficiently (6 to 14 times more than the free ON) taken up by liver cells when associated to lactosylated low-density lipoproteins, a lipid carrier, which is endocytosed by the galactose receptors expressed at the surface of hepatocytes *(9)*.

Despite these potential advantages, however, antisense ONs have mainly been administered in vivo by "brute force" up to now. This seemingly paradoxical situation might be explained in several ways.

First, delivery strategies are in their infancy, and a low cost, nontoxic, and efficient delivery vehicle for nucleic acids-based drugs is not yet available for preclinical or clinical studies. This situation is also encountered for gene transfer with nonviral vectors. Second, biological responses have been achieved with free antisense ON or ribozymes in animal models and in clinical trials.

Several strategies are being used routinely in laboratories to improve plasmid DNA tranfection or synthetic ON delivery (as reviewed in ref. *10*) but, unfortunately, most will be difficult to use in vivo.

Physical methods, such as electroporation and microinjection, are essentially limited to in vitro experiments. Electroporation, however, has been applied for in vivo plasmid DNA administration, at least in muscle cells.

Chemical methods as liposomes and cationic-lipids-based delivery systems are today more widely employed for the delivery of plasmid DNA and antisense ONs in most tissues. A main advantage of these strategies is to limit the degradation of the associated nucleic acids by nucleases in the biological fluids. Because liposomes are essentially taken up by endocytosis, escape from endocytic compartment and cytoplasmic delivery still remains a major limitation. Along this line, addition of a fusogenic peptide, as the peptide derived from the influenza hemaglutinin protein increases the efficiency of delivery *(11)*. Cationic lipids formulations are available on a commercial basis. Their use only requires mixing of the cationic lipids with the nucleic acid molecules in appropriate proportion.

The resulting positive charge of the complexes favors cell uptake by adsorptive endocytosis. Moreover, early escape from endocytic compartment seems to occur thus favoring cytoplasmic delivery (ref. *12* and references therein). However, the future of these formulations as transfection agents for in vivo experimentations will have to await long-term toxicity and bioavailability studies .

2. CELL-PENETRATING PEPTIDES: A SURVEY OF THEIR GENERAL PROPERTIES AND MAJOR APPLICATIONS

As summarized in the previous section, commonly used nonviral methods for nucleic acids delivery often capitalize on electrostatic interaction between the cationic delivery vehicle (poly L-lysine based conjugates, cationic liposomes, dendrimers, polythyleneimine, etc.) and negatively charged "receptors" at the cell surface. We will focus here on a new family of cationic delivery vehicles collectively known as cell-penetrating peptides (CPPs), whose prototype has been a basic peptide (penetratin) derived from the third helix domain of the Drosophila *Antennapedia* transcription factor.

These CPPs have been initially characterized by a high content in basic amino acids and by their ability to be rapidly internalized within most cell types by a mechanism that was initially claimed not to involve endocytosis (*see* Subheading 4).

We will review here major properties and applications of three of the most commonly used CPPs, namely penetratin, tat, and transportan.

2.1. Penetratin

Penetratin was discovered in attempts to understand the mechanism through which the Drosophila *Antennapedia* transcription factor was taken up by intact nervous cells. Cellular uptake was allocated to a short basic peptide (extending from amino acids 43 to 58) in the third helix of the *Antennapedia* protein *(13)*. Further structure-activity studies, including a systematic Ala scan mapping (in which each amino acid in the peptide has been replaced by an alanine residue), have concluded to the importance of hydrophobic (Trp in particular) and basic (Arg and Lys) residues for plasma membrane binding and subsequent cellular internalization *(14)*.

Along the same lines, a truncated version (Arg52-Arg-Met-Lys-Trp-Lys-Lys58) of penetratin was still able to cross the plasma membrane *(15)*. Surprisingly, the cellular uptake and nuclear translocation of penetratin still occurred at low temperature and did not appear to be saturable. Moreover retro- ,enantio- and inverso- analogues of the peptide were internalized as well. Altogether, internalization does not appear to involve binding to a chiral receptor and subsequent endocytosis. The mechanism of uptake has not been elucidated, although a model involving the formation of inverted micelles after binding to sialic acid residues (or to other negatively charged determinants) of the cell surface has been proposed (*see* ref. *16* for a review). Most interestingly, penetratin is able to carry various chemically conjugated cargoes within cells. These include antisense ON *(17)*, phosphopeptides interfering with signaling cascades (reviewed in ref. *18*), and doxorubicin to overcome multidrug resistance in cancer cells *(19)*. In the latter case, penetratin conjugation also led to increased delivery of doxorubicin across the blood–brain barrier *(20)*.

2.2. Transportan

Transportan is a 27 amino acids-long chimeric peptide in which the N-terminal portion of the neuropeptide galanin was coupled via a Lys residue to a fragment of the wasp venom toxin mastoparan. It is rapidly internalized in cells and translocated to the cell nucleus in a process that does not appear to involve endocytosis, as described for penetratins and for the tat peptide. It has been used as a synthetic vehicle for the delivery of various cargoes as well, but the most striking data have been obtained with peptide nucleic acids (PNAs) analog in an antisense approach, as detailed in Subheading 3. In an interesting recent study, a 3-nitrotyrosine quenching group was introduced in transportan (and in other cell-penetrating peptides). These modified peptide carriers were then conjugated through a disulfide bridge to a small peptide cargo carrying a fluorochrome. This elegant approach allowed to monitor unambiguously cellular uptake of the CPP-conjugated cargo. It was indeed verified that release of the fluorescent cargo required the reduction of the disulfide bridge, which occurs within cells only. Transportan appeared to be the most efficient transporter (as compared to tat and penetratin) at least for the small peptide cargo used in this model system. However, transportan induces significantly more membrane leakage than penetratin and tat, in parallel with its increased hydrophobic moment *(21)*.

2.3. Tat Peptide

The HIV-coded tat protein is an 86 amino acids-long nuclear protein that binds to the viral TAR region. It has been extensively studied by virologists for its ability to transactivate the HIV-promoter (*see* ref. *22* for a review). It became soon realized that incubation of cultured cells with the purified tat protein was sufficient to turn on the transcription of a reporter gene driven by the HIV promoter *(23)*. Further studies by several groups did confirm that the tat protein was internalized, most probably by endocytosis, and translocated to the nucleus. Moreover, the crosslinking of nonpermeant recombinant proteins as β-galactosidase to the basic domain of the tat protein (amino acids 37 to 72) allowed cellular uptake of these chimeric constructs in various cell lines *(24)*. These initial studies already pointed to the potential usefulness of tat-derived peptides as vehicles for the cellular delivery of chemically conjugated biomolecules.

At about the same time, as pointed out in Subheading 2.1, the translocation properties of another transcription factor, namely, the Drosophila *Antennapedia*, were assigned to the amphipathic character of a 16 amino acids-long region in the homeodomain third helix *(13)*.

Both sets of observations prompted studies in our group that aimed at delineating the shortest tat-derived peptide still able to cross efficiently the plasma membrane. The 37–72 region of tat encompasses two potentially important structural regions, namely, an N-terminal domain (from amino acids 39 to 49) that could adopt an amphipathic α-helix structure *(25)*, a central domain (amino acids 48 to 52) including a GRKKR nuclear localization signal, and a C-terminal basic region. A series of peptides including these various regions were chemically synthesized. The tat-derived peptides were conjugated through an additional C-terminal cysteinyl residue to a fluorochrome, and fluorescence distribution was analyzed on formaldehyde-fixed cells *(26)*. The intracellular distribution of tat has also been analyzed by indirect immunofluorescence with a monoclonal antibody specific to the tat basic domain.

These studies clearly established that the most efficiently internalized peptide encompassed the NLS signal, and the basic amino acids stretch but lacked the potential amphipathic helix. The NLS region was not sufficient since a peptide spanning the 37 to 53 region was not internalized. Along the same lines, amino acids substitutions in the *Antennapedia* peptide also ruled out the importance of the amphipathic α-helix for cellular uptake *(27)*.

A series of progressive deletions and amino acids substitutions (Ala scan mapping) then established the key role of all basic amino acids *(28)*. A 9-mer basic amino acids-rich tat sequence (Arg-Lys-Lys-Arg-Arg-Gln-Arg-Arg-Arg) thus appeared to be requested and sufficient for cellular uptake and nuclear translocation thus providing a first example, to our knowledge, of dual functions within a single short peptide.

As pointed in the introductory section, a major challenge in biotechnology is the design of vectors that will improve the cellular internalization of hydrophilic biomolecules. Our main strategy has consisted in the chemical conjugation of a cargo carrying an activated thiol function with the free sulfhydryl group of the cystein residue added to the C-terminal end of the tat-transporting peptide *(29)*. It is indeed assumed that the intracellular environment is reductive, thus allowing the intracellular release of a minimally modified cargo *(21)*. Nonpermeant peptides *(28)* and ON have been delivered this way. Alternatively, the transported biomolecule and the carrier tat peptide can be stably linked, through a peptide bond, for example.

Particularly interesting for cancer is the development of peptidic agonists or antagonists of intracellular signaling cascades and their vectorization through tat or *Antennapedia* CPP conjugation, as reviewed by Dunican and Doherty *(30)*.

Another promising application is the conjugation of the tat-basic peptide (sometimes called PTD, for protein transduction domain) to recombinant antigens, which leads to an impressive increase in cytotoxic T lymphocyte (CTL) responses, as demonstrated in a series of recent publications. As an example, a chimeric protein including the tat PTD and tumor-associated antigen was processed by dendritic cells and elicited an efficient CTL response in vivo after a single injection, thus providing an improved tool for cancer vaccine developments *(31)*.

In these experiments, conjugation through a reducible disulfide bridge or synthesis of a tandem peptide carrying contiguous cargo and transporting peptides have both been used. To our knowledge, no direct comparison of the biological response of the two approaches has been made in the same model in terms of efficiency and selectivity. Moreover, actual dissociation of the cargo peptide from its delivery vehicle has not been followed.

Somewhat unexpectedly, Dowdy and his colleagues *(32)* established that full-length proteins could be delivered into cells when carrying a fused tat basic domain (amino acids 47 to 57) at their N-terminal end in cell cultures or even in vivo after intraperitoneal injection into mice.

Allowing the cellular delivery of proteins by CPP fusion or conjugation offers many applications as reviewed by Ford et al. *(33)*. As a recent example, the site-specific Cre recombinase (which is a powerful tool for conditional mutagenesis and functional genomics in mammalian cells) has been fused to the tat peptide. The chimeric protein was efficiently translocated (with at least 50% efficiency) in all tested cell lines and primary cells (including murine embryonic stem cells and primary splenocytes which are difficult to transfect) as monitored by Cre-mediated recombination *(34)*.

Direct protein transduction and gene delivery have both limitations and advantages, and we will have to await more data before we will be able to appreciate their respective future and fields of applications.

Tat-conjugation even allows the intracellular delivery of particulate material. In a series of publications, biocompatible magnetic nanoparticles (with a mean diameter of several nanometers) were derivatized by tat peptides and their uptake in hematopoietic and neural progenitor cells for in vivo imaging purpose. Interestingly, conjugation of tat peptides to these superparamagnetic nanoparticles led to accelerated blood clearance and to increased accumulation in liver parenchyma, whereas untagged particles accumulated in endothelial and Kupffer cells (*see* ref. *35* and references therein).

Finally, tat peptides have been attached to the surface of liposomes (with a mean diameter of 200nm) via a polyethylene glycol spacer at an average of 500 tat-peptide per particle *(36)*. Cytoplasmic uptake of these large particles has been documented provided multipoint attachment between the tat-coated liposomes and the cell surface was allowed. Whether liposomes-encapsulated material will be released in the cytoplasm has not been established yet.

As mentioned above, structure-activity studies have pointed to the key role played by basic residues (and particularly by Arg residues). This has prompted several groups to investigate synthetic Arg-rich peptides (as Arg9) and guanidino peptoid derivatives as drug delivery vehicles (as reviewed in ref. 37).

3. TAT-MEDIATED DELIVERY OF NUCLEIC ACIDS AND RELATED MATERIAL

As mentioned in previous sections, the design of nonviral vectors for the efficient cellular internalization of nucleic acids is still a challenge. Cell-penetrating peptides represent a promising approach toward this goal.

In a first series of papers, Prochiantz and colleagues described the successful internalization in neurons of antisense ON that were conjugated to the *Antennapedia* peptide through a disulfide bridge. Inhibition of neurite outgrowth in vitro owing to the inhibition amyloid precursor protein synthesis *(17)* and cell death due to the down-regulation of Cu/Zn superoxide dismutase *(38)* were documented.

Along the same lines, the conjugation of an ON derivative carrying a pyridine sulfenyl-activated thiol function at its 5' end with the free sulfhydryl group of the cystein residue at the C-terminal end of the tat peptide allowed cellular internalization and nuclear delivery of the transported ON *(29)*.

Likewise, a 20-mer phosphorothioate ON analog complementary to the ribosome-binding site of the P-glycoprotein (P-gp) mRNA was conjugated to the tat peptide through a disulfide bridge *(39)*. Interestingly, the biological activity of this ON peptide conjugate was more efficient in the presence of serum at variance with most synthetic nucleic acids delivery vectors *(40)*. A specific inhibition of P-gp expression was attained at submicromolar concentration whereas much higher levels were required in the absence of a delivery vehicle in the same experimental model *(41)*. The same group recently reported efficient delivery of antisense ON conjugated to CPP (Antennapedia or tat) using an elegant approach in which the antisense ON corrected the splicing of an aberrant intron and allowed the expression of a reporter luciferase gene *(42)*.

PNAs are DNA mimics with promising pharmacologic properties because they have an unusually high metabolic stability and they hybridize in a sequence-specific way to complementary RNA or DNA with high affinity (*see* ref. *43* for a review. Despite their neutral backbone, they do not cross more efficiently biological membranes than negatively charged ON. Delivering unmodified PNAs remains a challenge because their uncharged backbone precludes most of the routinely used transfection strategies. It was first established that a PNA targeted to the translation region of prepro-oxytocin mRNA was rapidly internalized in neuronal cells when conjugated to a retro-inverso form of the *Antennapedia* peptide, thus plaiding for an absence of chiral requirement *(44)*.

Most impressively, a PNA oligomer complementary to the human galanin receptor type 1 mRNA was conjugated to penetratin or to transportan. The expression of galanin receptors in cultured cells and even in vivo after intrathecal administration in rats was down-regulated in a sequence-specific and dose-dependent manner *(45)*.

Along the same lines, the conjugation of a membrane active basic peptide (KFFKFFKFFK) to a short PNA complementary to ribosomal RNA led to a bactericidal effect that was around 100 times more efficient than with naked PNA *(46)*.

Altogether, CPPs appear as valuable tools for the administration of antisense ON and PNA even in an in vivo setting. This is particularly important since, as pointed earlier, very few synthetic nucleic acids delivery vehicles have yet proven to be useful in vivo.

4. MECHANISM OF CELLULAR UPTAKE AND NUCLEAR TRANSLOCATION

In their seminal paper, Mann and Frankel *(47)* established that the tat protein was internalized in HeLa cells by adsorptive endocytosis. Genetic and biochemical evidence for an involvement of cell surface heparan sulfate proteoglycans have recently be provided *(48)* although integrin receptors *(49)* and other cell surface determinants might be involved as well. Interestingly, heparan-sulfate-binding proteins share common characteristics with the tat basic domain, and mutations or modifications of arginine residues in this region inhibit tat uptake.

Whether cellular uptake of the tat peptide and of the other CPPs involve the same type of receptors has still to be firmly established. Along these lines, fluorochrome-labeled tat peptides were taken up in Chinese hamster ovary mutant cell lines deficient in the expression of heparan sulfate proteoglycans as monitored by fluorescence microscopy and by FACS scan analysis *(50)*.

CPP internalization did not appear to require specific cellular receptor/transporters. Tat and the other CPPs are efficiently taken up by most cell types including monocyte/macrophage progenitors, which are poorly transfected by traditional methods *(51)*. Moreover, tat peptide analogues assembled with *d*-amino acid derivatives *(inverso)* or synthesized from the C-terminal end to the N-terminal end (usually called *retro* sequence) *(52,53)* retained their ability to be internalized in cells.

It has been proposed that CPPs are rapidly taken up in cells at physiological and at low temperature by a mechanism that does not involve endocytosis or active transport *(see* ref. *54* and references therein). An interesting model has been proposed for penetratin that postulates the formation of inverted micelles between the positively charged peptide and the negatively charged membrane

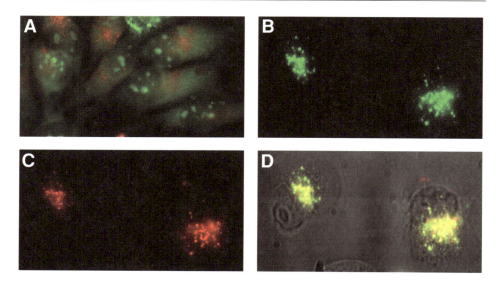

Fig. 1. Fluorescence microscopy micrographs of paraformaldehyde-fixed (**A**) and living unfixed (**B–D**) HeLa cells incubated with fluorochrome-labeled tat peptides. Cells were grown on coverslips and incubated for 20 min in the presence of Alexa 488-tagged tat48–60 peptide (**B**, green fluorescence) or Alexa 546-conjugated transferrin (**C**, red fluorescence). Upon coincubation, the two markers remain clearly distinct in fixed cells (**A**) whereas they predominantly colocalize in unfixed cells as attested by the resulting yellow fluorescence (**D**).

phospholipids, as reviewed in *(16)*. Experimental evidence has, however, remained scarce and controversial *(55)*.

More importantly, most studies on CPP uptake have made use of fluorescence microscopy on fixed cells and FACS analysis, in experimental conditions that can lead to artifacts.

Cell fixation, even in mild conditions with paraformaldehyde, leads to a dramatic redistribution of these peptides, as illustrated in Fig. 1.

As can be seen, tat peptide-associated fluorescence is diffused in the cytoplasm and largely concentrated in nucleoli in fixed cells, whereas it is predominantly vesicular in living unfixed cells, in keeping with an endocytic uptake mechanism.

Moreover, CPPs strongly bind to the cell surface. As a consequence, discriminating plasma membrane binding from cell internalization cannot be achieved unless a thorough washing step with proteases is introduced prior to FACS analysis *(56)*. Alternative strategies have been proposed, such as the use of NBD-labeled CPP whose fluorescence can be quenched by dithionite outside of the cell *(14)*. The mechanism of uptake of CPP is now being re-evaluated with these tools in several laboratories. Ongoing work in our group for tat and for Arg9 has already established that cellular uptake is a relatively slow energy-dependent process that most probably involves two steps, namely, binding to negatively charged cell surface components followed by internalization. The nature of these receptor(s) and the precise route followed by these CPPs and their conjugated cargoes are the object of ongoing studies.

REFERENCES

1. Crooke ST (ed). Antisense drug technology. New York: Marcel Dekker, 2001.
2. Faria M, Giovannangeli C. Triplex-forming molecules: from concepts to applications. J Gene Med 2001; 3:299–310.
3. Cho-Chung YS, Park YG, Lee YN. Oligonucleotides as transcription factor decoys. Curr Opin Mol Ther 1999; 1:386–392.
4. Sun LQ, Cairns MJ, Saravolac EG, Baker A, Gerlach WL. Catalytic nucleic acids: from lab to applications. Pharmacol Rev 2000; 52:325–347.
5. Bernstein E, Denli AM, Hannon GJ. The rest is silence. RNA 2001; 7:1509–1521.
6. Krieg AM. The role of CpG motifs in innate immunity. Curr Opin Immunol 2000; 12:35–43.
7. Degols G, Devaux C, Lebleu B. Oligonucleotide-poly(L-lysine)-heparin complexes: potent sequence-specific inhibitors of HIV-1 infection. Bioconjug Chem 1994; 5:8–13.
8. Juliano RL, Alahari S, Yoo H, Kole R, Cho M. Antisense pharmacodynamics: critical issues in the transport and delivery of antisense oligonucleotides. Pharm Res 1999; 16:494–502.
9. Bijsterbosch MK, Manoharan M, Dorland R, Waarlo IH, Biessen EA, van Berkel TJ. Delivery of cholesteryl-conjugated phosphorothioate oligodeoxynucleotides to Kupffer cells by lactosylated low-density lipoprotein. Biochem Pharmacol 2001; 62:627–633.
10. Akhtar S, Hughes MD, Khan A, et al. The delivery of antisense therapeutics. Adv Drug Deliv Rev 2000; 44:3–21.
11. Plank C, Oberhauser B, Mechtler K, Koch C, Wagner E. The influence of endosome-disruptive peptides on gene transfer using synthetic virus-like gene transfer systems. J Biol Chem 1994; 269:12918–12924.
12. Hafez IM, Maurer N, Cullis PR. On the mechanism whereby cationic lipids promote intracellular delivery of polynucleic acids. Gene Ther 2001; 8:1188–1196.
13. Derossi D, Joliot AH, Chassaing G, Prochiantz A. The third helix of the Antennapedia homeodomain translocates through biological membranes. J Biol Chem 1994; 269:10444–10450.
14. Drin G, Mazel M, Clair P, Mathieu D, Kaczorek M, Temsamani J. Physico-chemical requirements for cellular uptake of pAntp peptide. Role of lipid-binding affinity. Eur J Biochem 2001; 268:1304–1314.
15. Fischer PM, Zhelev NZ, Wang S, Melville JE, Fahraeus R, Lane DP. Structure-activity relationship of truncated and substituted analogues of the intracellular delivery vector Penetratin. J Pept Res 2000; 55:163–172.
16. Derossi D, Chassaing G, Prochiantz A. Trojan peptides: the penetratin system for intracellular delivery. Trends Cell Biol 1998; 8:84–87.
17. Allinquant B, Hantraye P, Mailleux P, Moya K, Bouillot C, Prochiantz A. Down regulation of amyloid precursor protein inhibits neurite outgrowth in vitro. J Cell Biol 1995; 128:919–927.
18. Dunican DJ, Doherty P. Designing cell-permeant phosphopeptides to modulate intracellular signaling pathways. Biopolymers 2001; 60:45–60.
19. Mazel M, Clair P, Rousselle C, et al. Doxorubicin-peptide conjugates overcome multidrug resistance. Anticancer Drugs 2001; 12:107–116.
20. Rousselle C, Clair P, Lefauconnier JM, Kaczorek M, Scherrmann JM, Temsamani J. New advances in the transport of doxorubicin through the blood-brain barrier by a peptide vector-mediated strategy. Mol Pharmacol 2000; 57:679–686.

21. Hallbrink M, Floren A, Elmquist A, Pooga M, Bartfai T, Langel U. Cargo delivery kinetics of cell-penetrating peptides. Biochim Biophys Acta 2001; 1515:101–109.
22. Jeang KT, Xiao H, Rich EA. Multifaceted activities of the HIV-1 transactivator of transcription, tat. J Biol Chem 1999; 274:28837–28840.
23. Frankel AD, Pabo CO. Cellular uptake of the tat protein from human immunodeficiency virus. Cell 1988; 55:1189–1193.
24. Fawell S, Seery J, Daikh Y, et al. Tat-mediated delivery of heterologous proteins into cells. Proc Natl Acad Sci USA 1994; 91:664–668.
25. Loret EP, Vives E, Ho PS, Rochat H, Van Rietschoten J, Johnson WC, Jr. Activating region of HIV-1 tat protein: vacuum UV circular dichroism and energy minimization. Biochemistry 1991; 30:6013–6023.
26. Vivès E, Brodin P, Lebleu B. A truncated HIV-1 tat protein basic domain rapidly translocates through the plasma membrane and accumulates in the cell nucleus. J Biol Chem 1997; 272:16010–16017.
27. Derossi D, Calvet S, Trembleau A, Brunissen A, Chassaing G, Prochiantz A. Cell internalization of the third helix of the Antennapedia homeodomain is receptor-independent. J Biol Chem 1996; 271:18188–18193.
28. Vivès E, Granier C, Prevot P, Lebleu B. Structure activity relationship study of the plasma membrane translocating potential of a short peptide from HIV-1 tat protein. Lettres In Peptide Science 1997; 4:429–436.
29. Vivès E, Lebleu B. Selective coupling of a highly basic peptide to an oligonucleotide. Tetrahedron Letters 1997; 38:1183–1186.
30. Dunican DJ, Williams EJ, Howell FV, Doherty P. Selective inhibition of fibroblast growth factor (FGF)-stimulated mitogenesis by a FGF receptor-1-derived phosphopeptide. Cell Growth Differ 2001; 12:255–264.
31. Shibagaki N, Udey MC. Dendritic cells transduced with protein antigens induce cytotoxic lymphocytes and elicit antitumor immunity. J Immunol 2002; 168:2393–2401.
32. Schwarze SR, Ho A, Vocero-Akbani A, Dowdy SF. In vivo protein transduction: delivery of a biologically active protein into the mouse. Science 1999; 285:1569–1572.
33. Ford KG, Souberbielle BE, Darling D, Farzaneh F. Protein transduction: an alternative to genetic intervention? Gene Ther 2001; 8:1–4.
34. Peitz M, Pfannkuche K, Rajewsky K, Edenhofer F. Ability of the hydrophobic FGF and basic TAT peptides to promote cellular uptake of recombinant Cre recombinase: a tool for efficient genetic engineering of mammalian genomes. Proc Natl Acad Sci USA 2002; 99:4489–4494.
35. Zhao M, Kircher MF, Josephson L, Weissleder R. Differential conjugation of tat peptide to superparamagnetic nanoparticles and its effect on cellular uptake. Bioconjug Chem 2002; 13:840–4.
36. Torchilin VP, Rammohan R, Weissig V, Levchenko TS. Tat peptide on the surface of liposomes affords their efficient intracellular delivery even at low temperature and in the presence of metabolic inhibitors. Proc Natl Acad Sci USA 2001; 98:8786–8791.
37. Rothbard JB, Kreider E, Pattabiraman K, et al. Arginine-rich molecular transporters for drugs: the role of backbone and side chain variations on cellular uptake. In: Langel U, ed. Cell penetrating peptides. Boca Raton: CRC Press; 2002:141–160.
38. Troy CM, Derossi D, Prochiantz A, Greene LA, Shelanski ML. Downregulation of Cu/Zn superoxide dismutase leads to cell death via the nitric oxide-peroxynitrite pathway. J Neurosci 1996; 16:253–261.
39. Hughes J, Astriab A, Yoo H, et al. In vitro transport and delivery of antisense oligonucleotides. Methods Enzymol 2000; 313:342–358.
40. Astriab-Fisher A, Sergueev DS, Fisher M, Shaw BR, Juliano RL. Antisense inhibition of P-glycoprotein expression using peptide- oligonucleotide conjugates. Biochem Pharmacol 2000; 60:83–90.

41. Alahari SK, Dean NM, Fisher MH, et al. Inhibition of expression of the multidrug resistance-associated P- glycoprotein of by phosphorothioate and 5' cholesterol-conjugated phosphoro-thioate antisense oligonucleotides. Mol Pharmacol 1996; 50:808–819.
42. Astriab-Fisher A, Sergueev D, Fisher M, Shaw BR, Juliano RL. Conjugates of antisense oligonucleotides with the tat and antennapedia cell-penetrating peptides: effects on cellular uptake, binding to target sequences, and biologic actions. Pharm Res 2002; 19:744–754.
43. Ray A, Norden B. Peptide nucleic acid (PNA): its medical and biotechnical applications and promise for the future. Faseb J 2000; 14:1041–1060.
44. Aldrian-Herrada G, Desarmenien MG, Orcel H, et al. A peptide nucleic acid (PNA) is more rapidly internalized in cultured neurons when coupled to a retro-inverso delivery peptide. The antisense activity depresses the target mRNA and protein in magnocellular oxytocin neurons. Nucleic Acids Res 1998; 26:4910–4916.
45. Pooga M, Soomets U, Hallbrink M, et al. Cell penetrating PNA constructs regulate galanin receptor levels and modify pain transmission in vivo. Nat Biotechnol 1998; 16:857–861.
46. Good L, Awasthi SK, Dryselius R, Larsson O, Nielsen PE. Bactericidal antisense effects of peptide-PNA conjugates. Nat Biotechnol 2001; 19:360–364.
47. Mann DA, Frankel AD. Endocytosis and targeting of exogenous HIV-1 tat protein. Embo J 1991; 10:1733–1739.
48. Tyagi M, Rusnati M, Presta M, Giacca M. Internalization of HIV-1 tat requires cell surface heparan sulfate proteoglycans. J Biol Chem 2001; 276:3254–3261.
49. Barillari G, Gendelman R, Gallo RC, Ensoli B. The tat protein of human immunodeficiency virus type 1, a growth factor for AIDS Kaposi sarcoma and cytokine-activated vascular cells, induces adhesion of the same cell types by using integrin receptors recognizing the RGD amino acid sequence. Proc Natl Acad Sci USA 1993; 90:7941–7945.
50. Silhol M, Tyagi M, Giacca M, Lebleu B, Vives E. Different mechanisms for cellular internalization of the HIV-1 tat- derived cell penetrating peptide and recombinant proteins fused to tat. Eur J Biochem 2002; 269:494–501.
51. Abu-Amer Y, Dowdy SF, Ross FP, Clohisy JC, Teitelbaum SL. TAT fusion proteins containing tyrosine 42-deleted IkappaBalpha arrest osteoclastogenesis. J Biol Chem 2001; 276:30499–30503.
52. Futaki S, Suzuki T, Ohashi W, et al. Arginine-rich peptides. An abundant source of membrane-permeable peptides having potential as carriers for intracellular protein delivery. J Biol Chem 2001; 276:5836–5840.
53. Wender PA, Mitchell DJ, Pattabiraman K, Pelkey ET, Steinman L, Rothbard JB. The design, synthesis, and evaluation of molecules that enable or enhance cellular uptake: peptoid molecular transporters. Proc Natl Acad Sci USA 2000; 97:13003–13008.
54. Langel U (ed). Cell penetrating peptides. Boca Raton: CRC Press 2002.
55. Gräslund A, Göran Eriksson LE. Biophysical studies of cell penetrating peptides. In: Langel U, ed. Cell penetrating peptides. Boca Raton: CRC Press 2002:223–244.
56. Richard JP, Melikor K, Vives E, Ramos C, Venbeure NB, Gait MJ, et al. Cell-penetrating peptides: a re-evaluation of the mechanism of cell uptake. J Biol Chem 2003; 278:585–590.

10 Molecular Vectors for Gene Delivery to Cancer Cells

Guy Zuber, PhD, Jean-Serge Remy, PhD, Patrick Erbacher, PhD, Pascale Belguise, PhD, and Jean-Paul Behr, PhD

1. INTRODUCTION

Cancer gene therapy relies on nucleic acid carriers. Because of their diversity, viruses fulfill most requirements for gene delivery in clinical situations. However, parallel evolution of viruses and their hosts has made foreign protein particles, as well as infected cells, effective targets for the immune system. Although the latter consequence can be turned into therapeutic benefit, the former excludes repetitive treatment, which is the only reasonable approach for a chronic disease such as cancer.

Artificial carriers can be developed without polypeptide components. They can even be coated with an inert layer, thus escaping most of the immune surveillance. Unfortunately, at best a few out of a billion copies of the gene reach the target cell nucleus. Unfavorable biodistribution, as well as ineffective intracellular trafficking, are responsible for this poor figure.

From: *Cancer Drug Discovery and Development:*
Nucleic Acid Therapeutics in Cancer
Edited by: A. M. Gewirtz © Humana Press Inc., Totowa, NJ

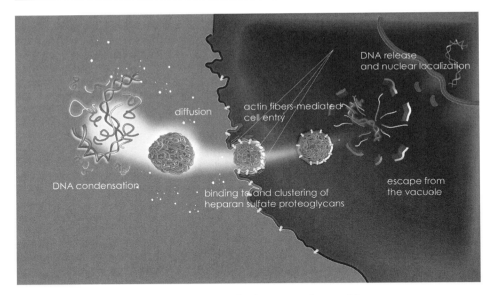

Fig. 1. Gene delivery with synthetic vectors is a multistep process.

2. SIZE OF THE DNA/CARRIER COMPLEXES

The course of a foreign gene to the nucleus of a cell is a complex multistage process that requires a multifunctional vector (Fig. 1). The core of synthetic vectors is invariably a polycation capable of inducing DNA condensation. Conversion of a filiform molecule into a compact particle improves both chemical stability and physical properties. Plasmid DNA compaction by cationic liposomes or polymers is a quasi-irreversible process that leads to microprecipitates containing hundreds of DNA molecules per particle. For transfection of cells in culture, large complexes are advantageous because they sediment onto the cells. Not unexpected, however, their in vivo transfection properties are weak because of size-restricted diffusion (among other causes).

Unlike the *poly*cationic species mentioned above, *oligo*cations such as spermine or cationic detergents interact with DNA reversibly. Equilibration ensures monodispersity, and entropy tends to direct the system toward the largest number of condensed DNA particles. As a consequence, each particle should be made of a single molecule of plasmid (i.e., the smallest possible particle). Unluckily, the other consequence of reversible binding is that DNA complexes do not withstand dilution or binding to polyanions, and hence cannot be used as DNA vectors *(1,2)*.

A chemical solution to this dilemma was found, based on *in situ* chemical conversion of the cationic detergent into a cationic lipid (Fig. 2) *(3)*. This two-step process, leading to monomolecular and stable DNA particles, was validated

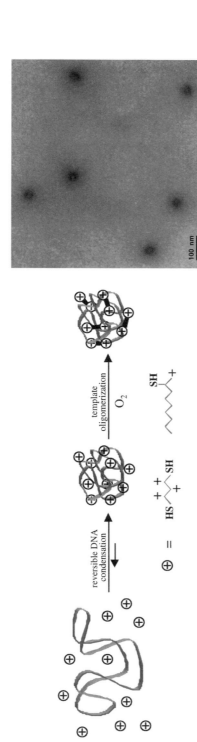

Fig. 2. DNA is condensed by thiol-containing oligocations presenting a low binding cooperativity. After equilibration, the particles are "frozen" by DNA template-assisted oxidation of thiols into disulfides. Transmission electron microscopy of the particles obtained from a 5.5 kbp plasmid shows a homogeneous population of 25-nm spheres.

131

using cysteine-based cationic detergents as condensing agents and thiol air oxidation into disulfide as the conversion reaction *(4)*. As shown in Fig. 2, the particles all have the same size (25 nm), which corresponds to the volume of a single molecule of plasmid DNA. Moreover, such particles are capable of moving through an agarose gel in electrophoresis conditions, in contrast to classical cationic lipid/DNA complexes, which remain in the wells. To our surprise, the particles moved even faster than plasmid DNA itself *(5)* (see also Fig. 4, lanes 1 and 5). Improved in vivo diffusion within tissues is thus expected. Intracellular trafficking may be favored, too, especially as noncondensed plasmid DNA was shown to be immobile in the cytoplasm *(6)*. Finally, the size of the particles remains compatible with active nuclear pore crossing, which may open the way to transfection of postmitotic cells.

3. CELL TARGETING AND ENTRY

To enter their hosts, many viruses and bacteria bind to cell/matrix- or cell/cell-anchoring proteins, such as heparan sulfate proteoglycans (HSPGs) and integrins. Anionic HSPGs are responsible for cell entry of species as different as chlamydia trachomatis *(7)*, adeno-associated virus *(8)*, and cationic proteins such as basic fibroblast growth factor *(9)* or TAT *(10)*. Interestingly, condensed DNA particles too require a cationic surface for gene delivery to be efficient *(11)*, and their cell entry was shown to be mediated by electrostatic interaction with HSPGs *(12–14)*. This is presumably true for all polycations, whether calcium phosphate-precipitated DNA or cationic peptide-tagged proteins and polynucleotides.

The cationic nature of all endocytosed species suggests a common mechanism for their cell entry. Among ubiquitous HSPGs that may act as receptors are the syndecans. These transmembrane proteins could cluster to form focal adhesions following individual electrostatic binding to a large polycationic entity. There is indeed evidence *(15)* that syndecan clustering induces binding to the actin cytoskeleton and eventually the formation of tension fibers. Yet tension would not provide mechanical stability to the cell, but rather the energy to engulf the cationic particle and form an intracellular vacuole (Fig. 1).

Unfortunately, in vivo a cationic DNA-containing particle immediately binds to circulating or extracellular matrix polyanionic proteins. This prevents most particles from reaching their target and eventually releases DNA from the complexes. In vivo, anionic proteoglycans are therefore too ubiquitous to serve as receptors for synthetic vectors. As discussed above, integrins share many functional properties with syndecans. Several integrins bind and internalize zwitterionic RGD peptide-presenting particles in vivo *(16)*. After the manner of adenovirus, RGD peptides were chemically conjugated to polycations such as polylysine *(17,18)* or polyethylenimine (PEI) *(19)* and complexed with DNA. The resulting particles were shown to deliver genes to epithelial cells in culture

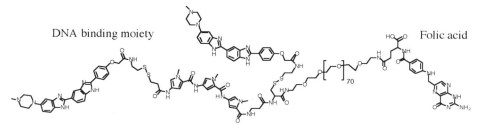

Fig. 3. Structure of the targeting element Z *bis*-(thio-[bisbenzimide])-tripyrole-PEG$_{3400}$-folate.

up to 100-fold better than the corresponding polycation/DNA complexes. Control experiment using RGE-coated particles confirmed the enhanced transfection to be due to $\alpha_v\,\beta_5$ integrin-mediated cell entry.

4. STEALTH PARTICLES

An attractive use of RGD-coated DNA particles would be targeting of the neovasculature of metastases following systemic delivery *(16)*. Indeed, resting endothelial cells of normal blood vessels express matrix-binding molecules at their basolateral side, whereas growing and less differentiated blood vessel cells of metastases express them also on the luminal side, hence the targeting. Intravenous injection experiments we performed with RGD-PEI/DNA complexes, however, did not target tumors better than the passive accumulation of PEI/DNA or transferrin–PEI/DNA complexes through the leaky vasculature *(20)*.

The biodistribution of widely different types of particles has been shown to benefit from coating with a layer of polyethyleneglycol (PEG). This effect is due to the inertness of the polyether backbone as well as to brush-type polymer crowding that prevents capture by macrophages. However, the latter physical property also prevents proper DNA condensation *(21,22)* and may also interfere with the DNA exchange/release process in the cell. PEI-PEG diblock polymers *(21,23,24)* or PEG post-grafting strategies *(25,26)* are being explored as a means to avoid interference with condensation.

As an example of combination of this approach with the monomolecular DNA particle technology discussed above, we currently attempt targeting *(27)* of the high-affinity folic acid receptor that is overexpressed on many cancer cells. Folic acid binding triggers internalization of the complexes. PEG (Mw = 3400) was conjugated to a strong DNA-binding moiety and to folic acid on the distal end (Fig. 3).

Monomolecular plasmid DNA particles were formed with a tetradecane-cysteine-ornithine detergent (C$_{14}$COrn) *(5)*. Aerobic disulfide bond formation led to stable (C$_{14}$COrn) $_2$/DNA complexes. Binding of Z to DNA as well as incorpo-

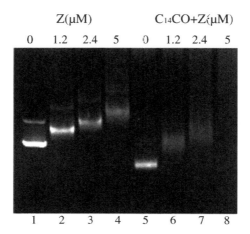

Fig. 4. Agarose gel electrophoresis shows binding of Z to plasmid DNA (compare lane 1 with lanes 2–4), formation of monomolecular DNA particles (lane 1 vs 5) as well as binding of Z to the particles (lane 5 vs 6–8).

ration of Z within the monomolecular DNA particles was monitored by gel electrophoresis (Fig. 4). Physicochemical measurements show particles coated with 2.4 μM Z to be compact, monomolecular, and stable in physiological conditions. Flow cytometry shows them to bind to KB cells (a human nasopharyngeal cancer cell line) when folate receptors are overexpressed (Fig. 5).

5. PROTON SPONGE-MEDIATED VACUOLE ESCAPE

After internalization, DNA complexes must escape from the formed intracellular vacuoles. Viruses that do not fuse at the plasma membrane exploit endosome acidification as an escape signal, by means of sophisticated conformational changes of fusion proteins. In the case of cationic lipids or polymer/DNA complexes, most particles probably remain trapped within the vacuoles. DNA being protected within the complexes, this may even be regarded as an effective "slow release" process.

Cationic lipids may possess some intrinsic bilayer-disrupting property, especially when forming nonlamellar phases (e.g., lipopolyamines form direct hexagonal phases [13]; DOPE forms an inverted one [28]). Subsequent vacuole rupture allows charge neutralization of the cationic lipid by intermixing with anionic phosphatidylserine from the vacuole outer leaflet. This may liberate in part the complexed polynucleotide (29).

Cationic polymers possess no fusogenic property *per se*. This is why fully cationized polymers such as polylysine require chloroquine, a lysosomotropic drug used to unmask the intravacuolar malaria parasite, to become effective

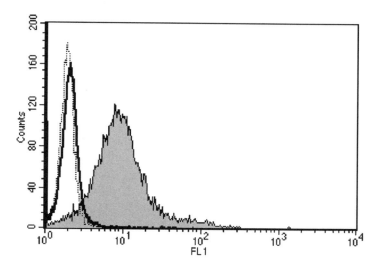

Fig. 5. Flow cytometry of KB cells incubated for 3 h with PEG_{3400}-folate monomolecular DNA particles (0.1% YOYO as fluorophore). Cells were grown in either folate-depleted (grey peak) or normal (bold line) cell-culture medium; dotted line: untreated cells.

transfection agents. However, cationic polymers *(30)*, such as polyamine dendrimers *(31,32)* or PEI *(33)*, share with chloroquine the ability to buffer the acidity of endosomes. The vacuolar pH should therefore decrease more slowly, with a large concomitant ionic concentration increase. Osmotic swelling due to water entry may then burst the vacuole and release the complex into the cytoplasm. This "proton sponge" hypothesis *(33)* proved to be fruitful, because it led to the design of other efficient polymeric vectors *(34–36)*. It was recently supported by the fact that PEI transfection efficiency is not further increased by chloroquine, but tremendously decreased by bafilomycin A, a specific vacuolar H^+-ATPase inhibitor *(37)*.

PEI, and especially linear PEI*(38)* is an attractive and versatile vector for in vitro and in vivo gene delivery. In the context of cancer therapy *(39)*, it has been used to deliver genes ex vivo to primary cultures *(40–42)*, as well as in animal models, by the intratumoral *(43)*, peritoneal *(44)*, topical *(45)*, aerosol *(46)*, and systemic *(20)* routes.

6. NUCLEAR MEMBRANE CROSSING

The largest barriers to gene delivery are restricted cytoplasmic diffusion and the nuclear membrane *(13,47)*. DNA particles entering fast dividing cells in culture are less confronted to these problems. Indeed, transfection of synchronized cells showed mitosis to be a key event for transfection to occur *(48,49)*. It

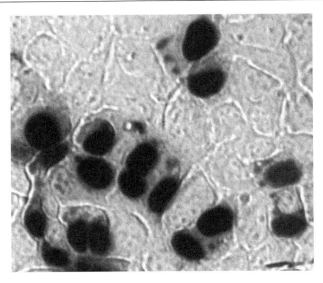

Fig. 6. BNL.Cl-2 hepatocytes transfected with nuclearLacZ/PEI complexes essentially appear as twins.

is therefore possible that DNA or DNA complexes that are unable to diffuse through the cytoplasm are dragged along with chromosomes and become incidentally sequestered in the nuclei of daughter cells during telophase. This would explain why most transfected cells appear as doublets (Fig. 6).

In vivo, even cancer cells can be considered as resting with respect to the lifetime of exogeneous DNA. A vectorial intracellular carrier must therefore be designed. Following the example of some DNA viruses, chemists attempt to divert the endogeneous nuclear import machinery by designing nuclear localization signal (NLS) peptide-bearing vectors (50–55). Unfortunately, cationic vector/DNA complexes are generally far too large to cross nuclear pores. Assuming the DNA/ cationic vector complexes are (at least in part) disassembled in the cytoplasm, we have covalently bound a single NLS peptide to one end of a linear DNA fragment. This hybrid construction was shown to enhance transgene expression up to 1000-fold (56). Our working hypothesis was that the 3-nm wide DNA–NLS molecules present in the cytoplasm would initially be translocated through a nuclear pore by the nuclear import machinery. As DNA enters the nucleus, it would be condensed into a chromatin-like structure, which would provide the mechanism for threading the remaining wormlike molecule through the pore.

7. CONCLUSION

Following the initial findings more than a decade ago that cationic lipids and polymers are able to carry genes into eukaryotic cells, much effort has been

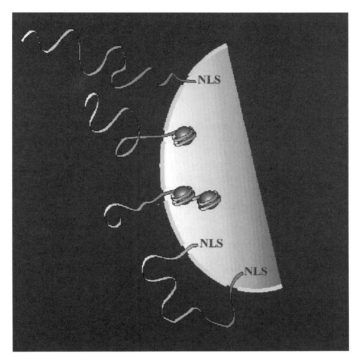

7. Nuclear pore crossing of a hybrid DNA–NLS peptide conjugate.

dedicated to improving transfection efficiency via structural modifications of the carrier. Exploiting structure/activity relations led to molecules capable to transfect adherent cell lines in culture at a multiplicity of infection of about 10^6 gene copies per cell. In vivo gene delivery, the prerequisite to gene therapy, is still orders of magnitude less effective.

Nowadays, nobody hopes anymore to discover the molecule able to carry DNA across the various barriers. Vectors of the future will be composed, much as viruses are, of multifunctional supramolecular systems that self-assemble around DNA. Programmed intracellular disassembly may well be part of a successful story, too. Each component of the vector is given a function. As illustrated above, some functions, such as integrin-mediated cell entry or NLS-directed entry into the nucleus, may just be mimicries of viruses. Some other solutions, such as monomolecular genome condensation via detergent dimerization, or endosome release by the proton sponge effect, have obviously not been exploited by the natural cell invaders. The consequences of increased complexity of the vectors on their development as gene medicines *(57)* are difficult to evaluate at this stage. In any case, the puzzle still has to be assembled prior to reassembling an artificial virus *(58)*—the quest of the Grail for the next decade?

REFERENCES

1. Remy JS, Sirlin C, Vierling P, Behr JP. Gene transfer with a series of lipophilic DNA-binding molecules. Bioconjug Chem 1994; 5(6):647–654.
2. Clamme JP, Bernacchi S, Vuilleumier C, Duportail G, Mely Y. Gene transfer by cationic surfactants is essentially limited by the trapping of the surfactant/DNA complexes onto the cell membrane: a fluorescence investigation. Biochim Biophys Acta 2000; 1467(2):347–361.
3. Blessing T, Remy JS, Behr JP. Template oligomerization of cations bound to DNA produces calibrated nanometric particles. J Amer Chem Soc 1998; 120:8519–8520.
4. Blessing T, Remy JS, Behr JP. Monomolecular collapse of plasmid DNA into stable virus-like particles. Proc Natl Acad Sci USA 1998; 95(4):1427–1431.
5. Dauty E, Remy JS, Blessing T, Behr JP. Dimerizable cationic detergents with a low cmc condense plasmid DNA into nanometric particles and transfect cells in culture. J Am Chem Soc 2001; 123(38):9227–9234.
6. Lukacs GL, Haggie P, Seksek O, Lechardeur D, Freedman N, Verkman AS. Size-dependent DNA mobility in cytoplasm and nucleus. J Biol Chem 2000; 275(3):1625–1629.
7. Su H, Raymond L, Rockey DD, Fischer E, Hackstadt T, Caldwell HD. A recombinant chlamydia trachomatis major outer membrane protein binds to heparan sulfate receptors on epithelial cells. Proc Natl Acad Sci USA 1996; 93(20):11143–11148.
8. Summerford C, Samulski RJ. Membrane-associated heparan sulfate proteoglycan is a receptor for adeno-associated virus type 2 virions. J Virol 1998; 72(2):1438–1445.
9. Quarto N, Amalric F. Heparan sulfate proteoglycans as transducers of FGF-2 signalling. J Cell Sci 1994; 107(Pt 11):3201–3212.
10. Tyagi M, Rusnati M, Presta M, Giacca M. Internalization of HIV-1 tat requires cell surface heparan sulfate proteoglycans. J Biol Chem 2001; 276(5):3254–3261.
11. Behr JP, Demeneix B, Loeffler JP, Perez-Mutul J. Efficient gene transfer into mammalian primary endocrine cells with lipopolyamine-coated DNA. Proc Natl Acad Sci USA 1989; 86(18):6982–6986.
12. Mislick KA, Baldeschwieler JD. Evidence for the role of proteoglycans in cation-mediated gene transfer. Proc Natl Acad Sci USA 1996; 93(22):12349–12354.
13. Labat-Moleur F, Steffan AM, Brisson C, et al. An electron microscopy study into the mechanism of gene transfer with lipopolyamines. Gene Ther 1996; 3(11):1010–1017.
14. Mounkes LC, Zhong W, Cipres-Palacin G, Heath TD, Debs RJ. Proteoglycans mediate cationic liposome-DNA complex-based gene delivery in vitro and in vivo. J Biol Chem 1998; 273(40):26164–26170.
15. Woods A, Couchman JR. Syndecan 4 heparan sulfate proteoglycan is a selectively enriched and widespread focal adhesion component. Mol Biol Cell 1994; 5(2):183–192.
16. Pasqualini R, Koivunen E, Ruoslahti E. Alpha v integrins as receptors for tumor targeting by circulating ligands. Nat Biotechnol 1997; 15(6):542–546.
17. Hart SL, Collins L, Gustafsson K, Fabre JW. Integrin-mediated transfection with peptides containing arginine- glycine-aspartic acid domains. Gene Ther 1997; 4(11):1225–1230.
18. Harbottle RP, Cooper RG, Hart SL, et al. An RGD-oligolysine peptide: a prototype construct for integrin-mediated gene delivery. Hum Gene Ther 1998; 9(7):1037–1047.
19. Erbacher P, Remy JS, Behr JP. Gene transfer with synthetic virus-like particles via the integrin-mediated endocytosis pathway. Gene Ther 1999; 6(1):138–145.
20. Kircheis R, Wightman L, Schreiber A, et al. Polyethylenimine/DNA complexes shielded by transferrin target gene expression to tumors after systemic application. Gene Ther 2001; 8(1):28–40.
21. Wolfert MA, Schacht EH, Toncheva V, Ulbrich K, Nazarova O, Seymour LW. Characterization of vectors for gene therapy formed by self-assembly of DNA with synthetic block copolymers. Hum Gene Ther 1996; 7(17):2123–2133.

22. Erbacher P, Bettinger T, Belguise-Valladier P, et al. Transfection and physical properties of various saccharide, poly(ethylene glycol), and antibody-derivatized polyethylenimines (PEI). J Gene Med 1999; 1(3):210–222.

23. Vinogradov S, Batrakova E, Li S, Kabanov A. Polyion complex micelles with protein-modified corona for receptor-mediated delivery of oligonucleotides into cells. Bioconjug Chem 1999; 10(5):851–860.

24. Kataoka K, Harada A, Nagasaki Y. Block copolymer micelles for drug delivery: design, characterization and biological significance. Adv Drug Deliv Rev 2001; 47(1):113–131.

25. Fisher KD, Ulbrich K, Subr V, et al. A versatile system for receptor-mediated gene delivery permits increased entry of DNA into target cells, enhanced delivery to the nucleus and elevated rates of transgene expression. Gene Ther 2000; 7(15):1337–1343.

26. Blessing T, Kursa M, Holzhauser R, Kircheis R, Wagner E. Different strategies for formation of pegylated EGF-conjugated PEI/DNA complexes for targeted gene delivery. Bioconjug Chem 2001; 12(4):529–537.

27. Gabizon A, Horowitz AT, Goren D, et al. Targeting folate receptor with folate linked to extremities of poly(ethylene glycol)-grafted liposomes: in vitro studies. Bioconjug Chem 1999; 10(2):289–298.

28. Lin AJ, Slack NL, Ahmad A, et al. Structure and structure-function studies of lipid/plasmid DNA complexes. J Drug Target 2000; 8(1):13–27.

29. Zelphati O, Szoka FC, Jr. Mechanism of oligonucleotide release from cationic liposomes. Proc Natl Acad Sci USA 1996; 93(21):11493–11498.

30. Demeneix B, Behr J, Boussif O, Zanta MA, Abdallah B, Remy J. Gene transfer with lipospermines and polyethylenimines. Adv Drug Deliv Rev 1998; 30(1-3):85–95.

31. Haensler J, Szoka FC, Jr. Polyamidoamine cascade polymers mediate efficient transfection of cells in culture. Bioconjug Chem 1993; 4(5):372–379.

32. Kukowska-Latallo JF, Bielinska AU, Johnson J, Spindler R, Tomalia DA, Baker JR, Jr. Efficient transfer of genetic material into mammalian cells using Starburst polyamidoamine dendrimers. Proc Natl Acad Sci USA 1996; 93(10):4897–4902.

33. Boussif O, Lezoualc'h F, Zanta MA, et al. A versatile vector for gene and oligonucleotide transfer into cells in culture and in vivo: polyethylenimine. Proc Natl Acad Sci USA 1995; 92(16):7297–7301.

34. Fajac I, Allo JC, Souil E, et al. Histidylated polylysine as a synthetic vector for gene transfer into immortalized cystic fibrosis airway surface and airway gland serous cells. J Gene Med 2000; 2(5):368–378.

35. Putnam D, Gentry CA, Pack DW, Langer R. Polymer-based gene delivery with low cytotoxicity by a unique balance of side-chain termini. Proc Natl Acad Sci USA 2001; 98(3):1200–1205.

36. Han S, Mahato RI, Kim SW. Water-soluble lipopolymer for gene delivery. Bioconjug Chem 2001; 12(3):337–345.

37. Kichler A, Leborgne C, Coeytaux E, Danos O. Polyethylenimine-mediated gene delivery: a mechanistic study. J Gene Med 2001; 3(2):135–144.

38. Brunner S, Furtbauer E, Sauer T, Kursa M, Wagner E. Overcoming the nuclear barrier: cell cycle independent nonviral gene transfer with linear polyethylenimine or electroporation. Mol Ther 2002; 5(1):80–86.

39. Schatzlein AG. Non-viral vectors in cancer gene therapy: principles and progress. Anticancer Drugs 2001; 12(4):275–304.

40. Ringenbach L, Bohbot A, Tiberghien P, Oberling F, Feugeas O. Polyethylenimine-mediated transfection of human monocytes with the IFN-gamma gene: an approach for cancer adoptive immunotherapy. Gene Ther 1998; 5(11):1508–1516.

41. Poulain L, Ziller C, Muller CD, et al. Ovarian carcinoma cells are effectively transfected by polyethylenimine (PEI) derivatives. Cancer Gene Ther 2000; 7(4):644–652.

42. Merlin JL, Dolivet G, Dubessy C, et al. Improvement of nonviral p53 gene transfer in human carcinoma cells using glucosylated polyethylenimine derivatives. Cancer Gene Ther 2001; 8(3):203–210.

43. Mahato RI, Lee M, Han S, Maheshwari A, Kim SW. Intratumoral delivery of p2CMVmIL-12 using water-soluble lipopolymers. Mol Ther 2001; 4(2):130–138.

44. Aoki K, Furuhata S, Hatanaka K, et al. Polyethylenimine-mediated gene transfer into pancreatic tumor dissemination in the murine peritoneal cavity. Gene Ther 2001; 8(7):508–514.

45. Lisziewicz J, Gabrilovich DI, Varga G, et al. Induction of potent human immunodeficiency virus type 1-specific T-cell- restricted immunity by genetically modified dendritic cells. J Virol 2001; 75(16):7621–7628.

46. Densmore CL, Kleinerman ES, Gautam A, et al. Growth suppression of established human osteosarcoma lung metastases in mice by aerosol gene therapy with PEI-p53 complexes. Cancer Gene Ther 2001; 8(9):619–627.

47. Zabner J, Fasbender AJ, Moninger T, Poellinger KA, Welsh MJ. Cellular and molecular barriers to gene transfer by a cationic lipid. J Biol Chem 1995; 270(32): 18997–19007.

48. Andreadis S, Fuller AO, Palsson BO. Cell cycle dependence of retroviral transduction: An issue of overlapping time scales. Biotechnol Bioeng 1998; 58(2–3):272–281.

49. Brunner S, Sauer T, Carotta S, Cotton M, Saltik M, Wagner E. Cell cycle dependence of gene transfer by lipoplex, polyplex and recombinant adenovirus. Gene Ther 2000; 7(5):401–407.

50. Remy JS, Kichler A, Mordvinov V, Schuber F, Behr JP. Targeted gene transfer into hepatoma cells with lipopolyamine-condensed DNA particles presenting galactose ligands: a stage toward artificial viruses. Proc Natl Acad Sci USA 1995; 92(5):1744–1748.

51. Sebestyen MG, Ludtke JJ, Bassik MC, et al. DNA vector chemistry: the covalent attachment of signal peptides to plasmid DNA. Nat Biotechnol 1998; 16(1):80–85.

52. Ludtke JJ, Zhang G, Sebestyen MG, Wolff JA. A nuclear localization signal can enhance both the nuclear transport and expression of 1 kb DNA. J Cell Sci 1999; 112(Pt 12):2033–2041.

53. Neves C, Byk G, Scherman D, Wils P. Coupling of a targeting peptide to plasmid DNA by covalent triple helix formation. FEBS Lett 1999; 453(1–2):41–45.

54. Ciolina C, Byk G, Blanche F, Thuillier V, Scherman D, Wils P. Coupling of nuclear localization signals to plasmid DNA and specific interaction of the conjugates with importin alpha. Bioconjug Chem 1999; 10(1):49–55.

55. Branden LJ, Mohamed AJ, Smith CI. A peptide nucleic acid-nuclear localization signal fusion that mediates nuclear transport of DNA. Nat Biotechnol 1999; 17(8):784–787.

56. Zanta MA, Belguise-Valladier P, Behr JP. Gene delivery: a single nuclear localization signal peptide is sufficient to carry DNA to the cell nucleus. Proc Natl Acad Sci USA 1999; 96(1):91–96.

57. Rolland AP. From genes to gene medicines: recent advances in nonviral gene delivery. Crit Rev Ther Drug Carrier Syst 1998; 15(2):143–198.

58. Nishikawa M, Huang L. Nonviral vectors in the new millennium: delivery barriers in gene transfer. Hum Gene Ther 2001; 12(8):861–870.

IV TARGETING

11 Considerations on the Design of Antisense Oligonucleotides

Rosel Kretschmer-Kazemi Far, *PhD*, Jens M. Warnecke, *PhD*, and Georg Sczakiel, *PhD*

CONTENTS

Dysregulated cellular gene expression may cause malignant cell proliferation in specific cases and, finally, may contribute to the development of cancer in man. Antisense oligonucleotides (asON) provide a tool to specifically interfere with aberrant, up-regulated, and viral gene expression. Thus, a causative therapeutic treatment of tumor development and tumor spread is conceivable in the use of asON provided that a molecular target, that is, a gene causatively related to tumor development is identified *(1–3)*. This is reflected by a number of clinical

From: *Cancer Drug Discovery and Development:*
Nucleic Acid Therapeutics in Cancer
Edited by: A. M. Gewirtz © Humana Press Inc., Totowa, NJ

studies in which asON are being investigated for their applicability and their therapeutic potential in cancer treatment *(4)*. Efficacy, necessary doses, and dose-dependent side effects of asON in humans are important issues that all are directly or indirectly related to the effectiveness of double-strand formation between the target RNA and the asON. This annealing step seems to be strongly influenced by the complex target structure and by characteristics of the asON sequence itself. It is desirable to understand those characteristics because the selection of favorable local target motifs along a long-chain target RNA crucially determines effectiveness of the corresponding asON in vitro and in vivo. Furthermore, assuming that once a lead asON has been identified and proven to be biologically active against a given target according to an "antisense mechanism," then the question of how close this case is to the maximally achievable inhibition arises. In this chapter, we address this issue and aim to discuss some relevant parameters and views on the design and the probability of success in the application of asON.

1. COMPUTER-PREDICTED TARGET STRUCTURES FOR HIGH-THROUGHPUT DESIGN OF EFFECTIVE asON

A number of experimental *(5–7)* and theoretical *(8–10)* approaches have been described by which asON can be designed at an increased probability of success when compared to a random selection of asON species against a given target *(11)*. One of the successful computational concepts that has been improved progressively *(12,13)* is described in the following paragraph and is schematically depicted in Fig.1

First, the target sequence is subdivided into overlapping segments of defined size and used to calculate low-energy secondary structures thereof. Local structural motifs that are assumed to represent favorable target structures for invading antisense strands are recorded, and their statistical likelihood to be adopted in vivo is evaluated in order to define promising local target sequences. In our experience such favorable targets should show a stretch of at least 8 to 10 consecutively unpaired nucleotides. When considering the influence of the software that is used to predict RNA structure, there is no systematic information available. However, in a comparison of our results of the identification of favorable local target sites for asON with the human ICAM-1 mRNA, by using either mfold version 2.0 or 2.3, revealed that, in sum, the frequency of success in the design of asON was similar, although some of the effective local targets were the same and others were different. At this preliminary stage we conclude that the version of mfold used here does not significantly influence the output.

In a second step, the nucleotide sequences of asON are being defined. To this, either the 5'- or the 3'- terminal sequences of the antisense strand are chosen such that they can anneal with a central portion of the unpaired local target structure.

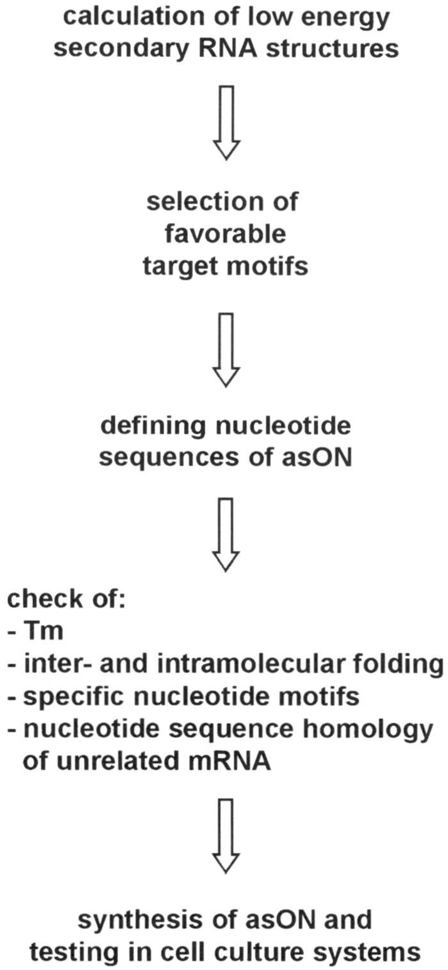

calculation of low energy
secondary RNA structures

selection of
favorable
target motifs

defining nucleotide
sequences of asON

check of:
- Tm
- inter- and intramolecular folding
- specific nucleotide motifs
- nucleotide sequence homology
** of unrelated mRNA**

synthesis of asON and
testing in cell culture systems

Fig. 1. Schematic depiction of a computational design of asON.

The total length of lead asON is usually between 18 and 20 nucleotides. Subsequently, specific characteristics of the asON species are checked. Properties that should be excluded are (i) a high potential of dimer formation and intramolecular folding *(14)*, (ii) a high degree of nucleotide sequence homology with unrelated transcribed sequences occurring in the targeted genome, and (iii) sequence motifs *(15)* including those that are known to cause undesired technical or biological effects, which include G-quartets or telomerase primer binding sites. Conversely, specific sequences are aimed to be included in the designed asON sequences as, for example, C-rich stretches are regarded as being related to high biological activity *(16,17)*. After having gone through this kind of filters only a relatively small portion of the initially chosen asON remain. Often this is in the order of 10 asON per 1000 nt of target sequence or less than that.

2. SUCCESS RATE OF THE THEORETICAL DESIGN OF ASON: WHAT IS THE MOST EFFECTIVE ASON MOLECULE IN THE RELEVANT SEQUENCE SPACE?

One of the fundamental open questions in the use of asON concerns the maximal extent of inhibition of target gene expression that is achievable by selecting the right asON sequence. In other words, how many asON species have to be tested to identify one that shows a given percentage of the hypothetically strongest asON inhibitor? The following considerations do not include the possibility to improve efficacy in living cells via parameters not related to target structure such as improved chemical modifications or improved modes of delivery.

Over recent years, the aforementioned approach to designing asON (Fig. 1) has been applied to a number of targets, including those listed in Table 1. Generally, it is assumed that 5 to 10% of all randomly chosen asON tested against a given target exert significant inhibition. Minimal significant inhibition of asON is often regarded as giving rise to 50% remaining gene expression on the level of mRNA or less than that. As a consequence the aim of different approaches to design effective asON can be defined as reducing the number of asON species to be tested to identify one that shows almost the efficacy in cell culture that can be maximally reached against a given target and at specific experimental conditions.

When comparing the results of the theoretical approach described here and experimental approaches to design asON, we feel that all are currently comparably successful. Major characteristics of different ways to design asON have been summarized recently *(11)*. However, there seem to be more options for further improvements of computational approaches, whereas experimental ways seem to have almost reached their limits.

To measure success we use the percentage of asON that is equal to or less than 50% expression of the target gene at reasonable asON concentrations. When considering the data shown in Table 1, keep in mind that the extent of asON-mediated inhibition is a sum of various parameters among which, we think, are local target structures and the characteristics of asON shown in Fig. 1.

The data summarized in Table 1 strongly suggest to use the strategy described in this work to select biologically active asON. From these data one might hypothesize that inducibly regulated gene expression is more sensitive to antisense inhibition than constitutively regulated gene expression. This is consistent with the observation that significant suppression of constitutive genes requires higher concentrations of asON than inducible ones.

Table 1. Examples for the Biological Activity of asON Designed According to the Scheme Described Here and Shown in Fig. 1.

Target	No. of asON	Conc. of asON (nM)	Detection level of gene expression	gene expression	total no. of asON[a]	Reference[b]
MMP2	21	400	RNA	Constitutive	4 (19%)	Sabelhaus et al., unpublished
Integrin $\alpha_v\beta_3$	12	50	RNA	Inducible	8 (67%)	Nedbal and Kronenwett, unpublished
ADAR1	8	100	RNA	Inducible	3 (38%)	Warnecke et al., unpublished
ICAM-1	57	100	Protein	Inducible	18 (32%)	Kretschmer-KF et al., in preparation
ICAM-1	37	100	Protein	Inducible	17 (46%)	12
HBV	3	50	Protein	Viral	2 (67%)	Unpublished

[a]Percentage of asON with inhibition ≥50%.
[b]Unpublished work from our laboratory.

3. WHAT DETERMINES OVERALL EFFICACY
OF ASON IN LIVING CELLS?

There seems to be a large set of biochemical and cellular parameters that influence the asON-induced phenotypic changes of a living cell. An antisense mechanism implies that the target is bound by asON sequence-specifically and in a dose-dependent way. Usually, this is accompanied by decreased levels of the target RNA; although in the case of local targets within the 5'-UTR or the ribosomal binding site, this is not always true. Furthermore, the gene product has to be suppressed, which should be causatively related to the phenotypic changes that are being observed. However, even if all of these requirements are fulfilled, in the case of successful asON-mediated knockout, one might have to deal with a mixed mechanism of action of the respective asON. For example, it is conceivable, and there is experimental evidence, that a given asON may exert a target- and sequence-specific antisense effect; a sequence-specific, non-antisense but target-specific suppressive effect; and a nucleotide sequence motif-specific (e.g., CpG) effect. It is anything but trivial to distinguish among such alternative modes of action, which may lead to the same or similar asON-induced phenotype. For example, a mixed mode of action seems to be the case for the bcl-2-directed asON G3139, which is in promising clinical trials in anticancer therapy.

4. ON THE RELATIONSHIP BETWEEN FUNCTIONAL
DOMAINS OF A TARGET mRNA
AND THE EFFICACY OF asON

However, one might speculate that there is a relationship between functional domains of a given target RNA and the extent of asON-mediated inhibition. Major functional domains of a mRNA include the 5'-UTR, the segment containing the translation initiation site including the start codon, the open reading frame, and the 3'-UTR, which in some cases is considered to influence mRNA stability and turnover. We addressed this hypothesis by comparing the number and percentage of effective asON directed against the various mRNA domains (Tables 2 and 3). Data from the literature and from our laboratory suggest that the coding sequence is the least favorable one, whereas the 5'-UTR and translational initiation site seem to allow asON-mediated inhibition at a relatively high success rate. Also, the 3'-UTR may be a favorable target in certain cases. For the translational start site, a high number of biologically active asON is found on the protein level (Table 2), which is not reflected on the level of target mRNA (Table 3). This could indicate that the effectiveness of asON against this functional domain does not necessarily require a RNase H activity, which seems to be important for the activity of asON against target domains located downstream.

A closer look at this issue is possible for ICAM-1 mRNA as a target because a large number of asON have been tested at comparable conditions in cell culture.

Table 2. "Hit Rate" of asON Related to mRNA Functional Domains
Monitored on the Level of Protein

5' UTR	TSS	CDS	3'-UTR	Reference
1/5	6/6	1/9	0/0	34
0/2	1/1	3/4	5/6	30
1/2	0/2	2/4	9/19	16
0/2	0/2	0/7	0/4	35
0/0	0/1	0/1	6/6	31
2/4	3/12	0/0	4/8	32
0/0	3/3	21/30	0/0	7
3/4	0/0	1/2	5/10	30
3/5	1/5	0/0	0/0	32
0/1	1/1	22/	4/5	28
0/0	3/4	1/5	0/10	29
9/11	3/5	5/5	3/5	32
0/0	1/3	9/31	1/3	12
0/0	3/3	6/67	2/14	Unpublished[*]
Total: 19/36	25/48	51/167	39/90	
53%	52%	31%	43%	

TSS, translational start site including 10 nt upstream and 10 nt downstream of the start codon; CDS, coding sequence; *, unpublished data from our laboratory.

Table 3. "Hit Rate" of asON Related to mRNA Functional Domains
Monitored on the Level of RNA

5'-UTR	TSS	CDS	3'-UTR	Reference
4/9	1/2	0/1	4/20	33
0/1	0/4	0/5	6/13	36
0/0	0/0	13/63	0/0	Unpublished[*]
0/0	0/3	5/8	3/4	Unpublished[*]
Total: 4/10	1/9	18/77	13/37	
40%	11%	23%	35%	

TSS, translational start site including 10 nt upstream and 10 nt downstream of the start codon; CDS, coding sequence; *, unpublished data from our laboratory.

This analysis indicates a high degree of significant inhibition when the 5'-UTR/ AUG-segment or the 3'-portion of the open reading frame and the upstream portion of the 3'-UTR are directed by asON (Fig. 2). Conversely, most parts of the open reading frame and the downstream portion of the 3'-UTR seem to represent unfavorable targets in the case of this target. It is noteworthy, however, that here we look at the spliced form of the ICAM-1 mRNA. For this reason one cannot derive information on the role of intron sequences and exon/intron boundaries as functional domains directed by asON.

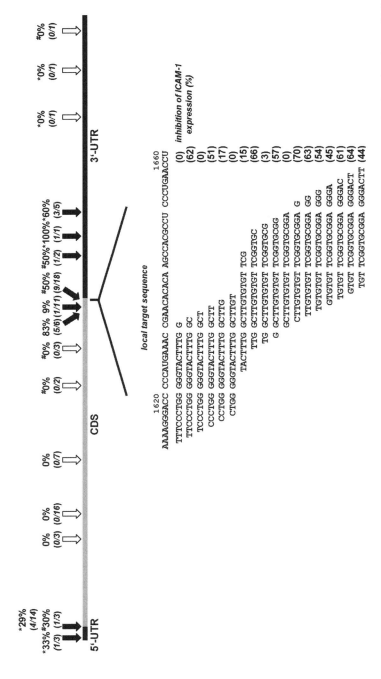

Fig. 2. Relationship between the effectiveness of ICAM-1-directed asON, the percentage and total numbers of asON that show≥50% inhibition in cell culture, and local functional domains of the spliced target mRNA (upper panel). The lower panel shows the high variability of biological activity of related asON directed against one local target segment between sequence positions 1620 and 1660 of the target. Abbreviations: *, data derived from ref. 32; #, data derived from ref. 12. Favorable local targets are indicated by filled arrows, unfavorable ones are indicated by open arrows.

150

5. THE ACTION OF asON: WHAT IS DIFFERENT BETWEEN A BUFFER IN VITRO AND A LIVING CELL?

The question is frequently asked whether all the biochemical analyses and identified rules governing the recognition and double-strand formation between complementary nucleic acids in vitro are really relevant for the situation inside a living cell, in particular, inside a mammalian cell. In this section several arguments (although not a complete list) will be summarized that indicate a meaningful relationship between the annealing reaction in a test tube and in living cells.

One might speculate that the formation of secondary and tertiary structure of long-chain target RNA could be sensitive to its biochemical environment, and hence, the annealing between complementary RNA strands could be different in cells versus inorganic buffer in vitro. A very sensitive monitor system to this possibility is the annealing step between two complementary RNA strands.

First, RNA–RNA annealing is thought to be increased intracellularly by facilitators, including the hnRNP protein A1 *(18)* for which the cationic detergent cetyltrimethylammonium bromide (CTAB) serves as a defined organic model compound *(19,20)*. Similarly, p53 was shown to bind to RNA and to promote the annealing of complementary RNA strands *(21–23)*. All of those molecules increase the kinetics of the annealing of long-chain RNA by two to three orders of magnitude in vitro. When probing the structure of RNA at conditions at which facilitators bind to RNA and of maximal facilitated annealing, there is no measurable evidence for facilitator-mediated changes of RNA structure. This was shown by various means including chemical and enzymatic probing, temperature gradient gel electrophoresis, and circular dichroism studies *(23,24)*. These findings suggest that compounds that bind to RNA and increase the annealing kinetics do not necessarily alter RNA structures and work as RNA "chaperones." Neither is it necessary to assume different annealing mechanisms in vitro and in vivo to explain increased annealing kinetics.

Another piece of evidence is related to the observation that sets of homologous derivatives of biologically active RNAs show a clear structure–function relationship that is related to RNA structures resolved in vitro, which include, for example, the natural system copA/copT in bacteria *(25)* and the effective HIV-1-directed antisense RNA αY69 *(26)*. The proposed pairing mechanisms critically involve structural motifs of the RNAs and are compatible with the structural models as well as with the activity of such families of derivatives in vivo and in living mammalian cells, respectively. This is no proof of altered RNA structures inside cells versus the in vitro situation, and there is no necessity to assume such differences.

Finally, when looking at the binding of asON with structured target RNA, there is another line of evidence suggesting a great similarity of the annealing in vitro and in living cells. When assuming that the complex relationship among

RNA structure, annealing kinetics, and biological activity is highly sensitive to structural changes of the target, then the structure-annealing relationship in vitro and the relationship between annealing and biological activity in cells should not be consistent in case of significant structural differences. However, one observes an obvious correlation among structure-dependent parameters, the annealing kinetics, and the biological activity of asON in case of asON directed against the human papillomavirus type 16 *(27)*.

6. PROSPECTS

Future improvements of the effectiveness of asON in living cells and in vivo, however, should also include parameters that are not related to the function and structure of the target RNA. It seems to be promising to consider new concepts and approaches to the mode of delivery desirably in a cell type or tissue-specific way, the specific nucleic acid chemistry used, and the combination of antisense mechanisms with other mechanisms of target gene suppression such as those including catalytic modes of action.

ACKNOWLEDGMENTS

We thank A. Hopert for critical comments on this manuscript. This work was supported by the "Deutsche Forschungsgemeinschaft" (grant no. Sc14/1-3) and the "Forschungsschwerpunkt Onkologie" of the University of Lübeck.

REFERENCES

1. Jen KY, Gewirtz AM. Suppression of gene expression by targeted disruption of messenger RNA: available options and current strategies. Stem Cells. 2000;18:307–319.
2. Crooke ST. Basic principles of antisense technology. In: Antisense drug technology: principles, strategies, and applications, ed. Marcel Dekker, New York, 2001:1–28.
3. Tamm I, Dörken B, Hartmann G. Antisense therapy in oncology: new hope for an old idea? Lancet 2002; 358:489–497.
4. Yuen AR, Sikic BI. Clinical studies of antisense therapy in cancer. Front Biosci 2000; 5:D588–593.
5. Milner N, Mir KU, Southern EM. Selecting effective antisense reagents on combinatorial oligonucleotide arrays. Nat Biotechnol 1997; 15:537–541.
6. Lima WF, Brown-Driver V, Fox M, Hanecak R, Bruice TW. Combinatorial screening and rational optimization for hybridization to folded hepatitis C virus RNA of oligonucleotides with biological antisense activity. J Biol Chem 1997; 272:626–638.
7. Ho SP, Bao Y, Lesher T, Malhotra R, Ma LY, Fluharty SJ, Sakai RR. Mapping of RNA accessible sites for antisense experiments with oligonucleotide libraries. Nat Biotechnol 1998; 16:59–63.
8. Mathews DH, Burkard ME, Freier SM, Wyatt JR, Turner DH. Predicting oligonucleotide affinity to nucleic acid targets. RNA 1999; 5:1458–1469.
9. Amarzguioui M, Brede G, Babaie E, Grotli M, Sproat B, Prydz H. Secondary structure prediction and in vitro accessibility of mRNA as tools in the selection of target sites for ribozymes. Nucleic Acids Res 2000; 28:4113–4124.

10. Ding Y, Lawrence CE. Statistical prediction of single-stranded regions in RNA secondary structure and application to predicting effective antisense target sites and beyond. Nucleic Acids Res 2001; 29:1034–1046.

11. Sczakiel G. Theoretical and experimental approaches to design effective antisense oligonucleotides. Front Biosci 2000; 5:194–201.

12. Patzel V, Steidl U, Kronenwett R, Haas R, Sczakiel G. A theoretical approach to select effective antisense oligodeoxyribonucleotides at high statistical probability. Nucleic Acids Res 1999; 27:4328–4334.

13. Kretschmer-Kazemi Far R, Nedbal W, Sczakiel G. Concepts to automate the theoretical design of effective antisense oligonucleotides. Bioinformatics 2001; 17:1058–1061.

14. Mitsuhashi M. Strategy for designing specific antisense oligonucleotide sequences. J Gastroenterol 1997; 32:282–287.

15. Smetsers TF, Boezeman JB, Mensink EJ. Bias in nucleotide composition of antisense oligonucleotides. Antisense Nucleic Acid Drug Dev 1996; 6:63–67.

16. Tu GC, Cao QN, Zhou F, Israel Y. Tetranucleotide GGGA motif in primary RNA transcripts. Novel target site for antisense design. J Biol Chem 1998; 273:25125–25131.

17. Matveeva OV, Tsodikov AD, Giddings M, et al. Identification of sequence motifs in oligonucleotides whose presence is correlated with antisense activity. Nucleic Acids Res 2000; 28:2862–2865.

18. Pontius BW, Berg P. Renaturation of complementary DNA strands mediated by purified mammalian heterogeneous nuclear ribonucleoprotein A1 protein: implications for a mechanism for rapid molecular assembly. Proc Natl Acad Sci USA 1990; 87:8403–8407.

19. Pontius BW, Berg P. Rapid renaturation of complementary DNA strands mediated by cationic detergents: a role for high-probability binding domains in enhancing the kinetics of molecular assembly processes. Proc Natl Acad Sci USA 1991; 88:8237–8241.

20. Pontius BW. Close encounters: why unstructured, polymeric domains can increase rates of specific macromolecular association. Trends Biochem Sci 1993; 18:181–186.

21. Oberosler P, Hloch P, Ramsperger U, Stahl H. p53-catalyzed annealing of complementary single-stranded nucleic acids. EMBO J 1993; 12:2389–2396.

22. Wu L, Bayle JH, Elenbaas B, Pavletich NP, Levine AJ. Alternatively spliced forms in the carboxy-terminal domain of the p53 protein regulate its ability to promote annealing of complementary single strands of nucleic acids. Mol Cell Biol 1995; 15:497–504.

23. Nedbal W, Frey M, Willemann B, Zentgraf H-W, Sczakiel G. Mechanistic insights into p53-promoted RNA-RNA annealing. J Mol Biol 1997; 266:677–687.

24. Nedbal W, Homann M, Sczakiel G. The association of complementary ribonucleic acids can be greatly increased without lowering the Arrhenius activation energy or significantly altering RNA structure. Biochemistry 1997; 36:13552–13557.

25. Wagner EG, Simons RW. Antisense RNA control in bacteria, phages, and plasmids. Annu Rev Microbiol 1994; 48:713–742.

26. Eckardt S, Romby P, Sczakiel G. Implications of RNA structure on the annealing of a potent antisense RNA directed against the human immunodeficiency virus type 1. Biochemistry 1997; 36:12711–12721.

27. Venturini F, Braspenning J, Homann M, Gissmann L, Sczakiel G. Kinetic selection of HPV-16 E6/E7-directed antisense nucleic acids: anti-proliferative effects on HPV 16-transformed cells. Nucleic Acids Res 1999; 27:1585–1592.

28. Chiang MY, Chan H, Zounes M.A, Freier SM, Lima WF, Bennett CF. Antisense oligonucleotides inhibit intercellular adhesion molecule 1 expression by two distinct mechanisms. J Biol Chem 1991; 266:18162–18171.

29. Dean NM, McKay R, Condon TP, Bennett CF. Inhibition of protein kinase C-alpha expression in human A549 cells by antisense oligonucleotides inhibits induction of intercellular adhesion molecule 1 (ICAM-1) mRNA by phorbol esters. J Biol Chem 1994; 269:16416–16424.

30. Bennett CF, Condon TP, Grimm S, Chan H, Chiang MY. Inhibition of endothelial cell adhesion molecule expression with antisense oligonucleotides. J Immunol 1994; 152:3530–3540.
31. Stepkowski SM, Tu Y, Condon TP, Bennett CF. Blocking of heart allograft rejection by intercellular adhesion molecule-1 antisense oligonucleotides alone or in combination with other immunosuppressive modalities. J Immunol 1994; 153:5336–5346.
32. Lee CH, Chen HH, Hoke G, Jong JS, White L, Kang YH. Antisense gene suppression against human ICAM-1, ELAM-1, and VCAM-1 in cultured human umbilical vein endothelial cells. Shock 1995; 4:1–10.
33. Monia BP, Johnston JF, Geiger T, Muller M, Fabbro D. Antitumor activity of a phosphorothioate antisense oligodeoxynucleotide targeted against C-raf kinase. Nature Med 1996; 2:668–675.
34. Ho SP, Britton DH, Stone BA, et al. Potent antisense oligonucleotides to the human multidrug resistance-1 mRNA are rationally selected by mapping RNA-accessible sites with oligonucleotide libraries. Nucleic Acids Res 1996; 24:1901–1907.
35. Stewart AJ, Canitrot Y, Baracchini E, Dean NM, Deeley RG, Cole SP. Reduction of expression of the multidrug resistance protein (MRP) in human tumor cells by antisense phosphorothioate oligonucleotides. Biochem Pharmacol 1996; 51:461–469.
36. Miraglia L, Geiger T, Bennett CF, Dean NM. Inhibition of interleukin-1 type I receptor expression in human cell-lines by an antisense phosphorothioate oligodeoxynucleotide. Int J Immunopharmacol 1996; 18:227–240.

12 Identification of Hybridization Accessible Sequence in Messenger RNA

Lida K. Gifford, PhD, Ponzy Lu, PhD, and Alan M. Gewirtz, MD

CONTENTS

1. INTRODUCTION

A major obstacle to employing short complementary nucleic acid strands for modulating gene expression is the apparent randomness with which target mRNAs are inhibited *(1)*. We have hypothesized that the inability to predict mRNA structure in vivo is a significant component of this problem because it is not known which regions of an mRNA molecule are accessible for basepairing or other recognition processes. A number of strategies have been developed to ask if a region of mRNA is single-stranded and free of bound protein, but all have their limitations. Accordingly, we have attempted to develop a different approach to this problem.

To locate single-stranded accessible regions in an RNA molecule, we sought to develop probes that would allow us to visualize hybridization of an antisense nucleic acid with its mRNA target in vitro and in vivo. To this end, we have developed fluorescence-based self-quenching reporter molecules (SQRM),

From: *Cancer Drug Discovery and Development:*
Nucleic Acid Therapeutics in Cancer
Edited by: A. M. Gewirtz © Humana Press Inc., Totowa, NJ

based in part on the work of Tyagi and Kramer, who first reported the use of labeled DNA stem loops, which they called molecular beacons, that would only signal upon hybridization with their complementary target *(2)*. These molecules have found use in a variety of assays, but in particular for real-time PCR employed for molecular diagnosis. We recently showed that such molecules could be used for real-time, in vivo imaging of DNA/RNA hybridization *(3)* and have now extended their use to mapping hybridization accessible sites on mRNA.

2. DESIGN AND BIOPHYSICAL CHARACTERIZATION OF SQRM

As previously reported *(3)*, we synthesized SQRM molecules with 34-nucleotide (nt) stem-loop structure composed of 5-nt complementary flanking sequences and a 24-nt intervening loop sequence (Fig. 1). EDANS, the fluorescent donor, and DABCYL, the acceptor, were conjugated to the 5' and 3' ends of the molecule, respectively. Theoretically, when the SQRM is in the stem-loop configuration, the EDANS and DABCYL moieties are in close enough proximity so that direct collisional quenching, as well as FRET, occurs, and as a result, the molecules can emit no fluorescence. In the presence of a complementary target sequence, a bimolecular helix is formed, causing the stem loop to open. The fluorophore and quenching moieties then move far enough apart in space so that quenching interactions are negated, and a detectable signal may then be emitted upon excitation of the fluorescence donor group. To test this prediction, SQRM with different loop sequences were mixed in solution with a variety of oligonucleotide target sequences, excited by ultraviolet light (336 nm peak wavelength) and then examined with a spectrofluorometer for the emission signal. As expected, fluorescence signal was detected only when SQRM were placed in solution with ogliodeoxynucleotide (ODN) target to which they could hybridize.

Using serial dilutions of preformed SQRM/ODN duplexes microinjected into K562 cells, we found that we could detect as little approx 10 molecules of SQRM per cell. If the average cell is approx 10^{-12}–10^{-11} liters, we calculated that we should be able to detect approx 20–200 pM RNA. Based on these calculations, we hypothesized that we would be able to detect SQRM–mRNA hybridization, real time, in living cells. We tested this prediction by microinjecting 150 μM solutions of AS or SCR (control) SQRM into living K562 human leukemia cells. After injection, the cells were examined for signal by phase and fluorescence microscopy (Fig. 2). Higher levels of cellular fluorescence were observed in cells injected with AS SQRM (Fig. 2C,D) than those injected with control SQRM (Fig. 2A,B). Uninjected cells displayed no discernible fluorescence (Fig. 2E,F). Specificity of the fluorescence signal was further determined by injecting fibroblasts with the same SQRM. Because these cells do not express the mRNA to which the SQRM were targeted, they gave no fluorescence.

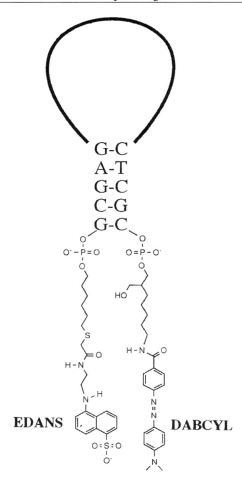

Fig. 1. Molecular beacon (SQRM) structure. SQRMs were synthesized as described with a 24 nucleotide "loop" sequence flanked on the 5' and 3' ends with complementary sequence 5 nucleotides long. Internal hybridization of the complementary ends creates the stem-loop structure. The fluorescent donor (EDANS) and acceptor (DABCYL) molecules are joined to the 5' terminal phosphate, and the 3' terminal hydroxyl group, respectively, through —(CH2)6—S—CH2—CO and —(CH2)7—NH linker arms. (Adapted from ref. *3*.)

We quantified the intensity of fluorescent signals emitted from SQRM–mRNA duplexes by using image analysis software. Fluorescence intensity of antisense SQRM complexed to target mRNA was approx 2.2-fold higher than sequence matched controls relative to a manufactured fluorescent standard. The fluorescence intensity of AS-SQRM targeting β-actin sequences was approx 5.5-fold higher than matched controls. This result was anticipated because β-actin mRNA

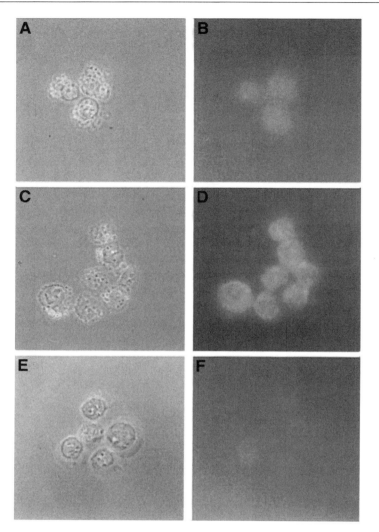

Fig. 2. Fluorescence emission in cells after SQRM microinjection. Fluorescence emission of SQRM after microinjection into K562 hematopoietic cells: After injection of 150 μ*M* solutions of vav AS or SCR (control) SQRM into living K562 human leukemia cells, the cells were examined for signal by phase (A, C, and E) and corresponding fluorescence (B, D, and F, respectively) microscopy. Significantly higher levels of cellular fluorescence were observed in cells injected with antisense SQRM (C and D) than those injected with SCR SQRM (A and B). Uninjected cells displayed no fluorescence (E and F). Panel A shows uninjected control cells photographed under phase, B is the corresponding fluorescent photomicrograph. C and E are antisense-SQRM– and SCR-SQRM–injected K562 cells, respectively, photographed under phase, whereas D and F are their corresponding fluorescent counterparts, respectively. Note that maximal fluorescent emission is found in antisense-SQRM-injected cells.

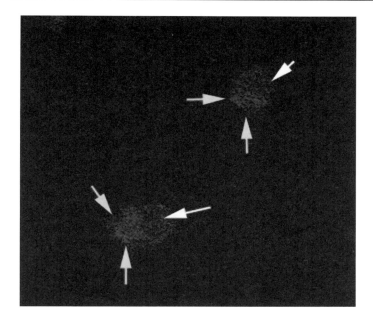

Fig. 3. Confocal image of K562 cells injected with antisense (as) vav SQRM. Cells injected with as vav SQRM revealed fluorescence signal when irradiated by a laser tuned to excite at 351nm. Fluorescence images were gathered approx15–30 min after SQRM injection and appeared stronger in the cells' cytoplasm (outlined by gray arrows) than in the nucleus (white arrow) suggesting that hybridization may be favored in the latter location. Uninjected cells, or cells injected with control SQRM, displayed little or no signal and were therefore very dark or unseen.

is expressed at higher copy number than vav. Approximately 50 cells were injected with either AS or control SQRM and examined for fluorescence emission within each experiment. The experiment was repeated three times, and data reported as mean ±SD.

We then attempted to more finely localize the intracellular location(s) of SQRM–mRNA duplex formation using confocal microscopy. AS and control SQRM were injected into living cells, which were then examined as described in the methods (Fig. 3). Little or no signal was observed in cells injected with control (SCR sequence) SQRM (not shown). In contrast, cells injected with AS vav SQRM revealed fluorescence signal when irradiated by a laser tuned to excite at 351 nm (Fig. 3). Considerably more fluorescence was observed in the area corresponding to the cell's cytoplasm than nucleus, suggesting that hybridization was favored in the latter location.

To gain an appreciation of the time course of hybridization between vav-targeted AS SQRMs and their mRNA target, we microinjected SQRMs into approx 100 K562 cells under direct microscopic visualization using a microma-nipulator. All injections were accomplished within approx 14 min after which time the slides were coverslipped and illuminated with ultraviolet (UV) light for 50 s. The slides were then viewed with a fluorescence microscope equipped with UV fluoride lenses. Fluorescence was easily detectable in the AS SQRM injected cells, whereas none was observed in cells injected with control SQRM. Accord-ingly, these experiments indicate that the injected SQRMs find and hybridize with their endogenous mRNA target within 15 min of being introduced into the cell.

In additional experiments we noted that control SQRM exposed to constant UV light also emitted fluorescent signals after approx 45 min of excitation. This suggested that intracellular nucleases may have degraded the SQRM hairpin-loop structure or that transient opening or "breathing" of the SQRM molecule was occurring. Either explanation is possible because fluorescence would not be observed in SQRMs that maintained their predicted conformation. Of interest, the apparent degradation of SQRM/target duplexes over time can be used to estimate the half-life of the SQRM in an intracellular environment. From exami-nation of more than 800 cells within eight separate experiments, phosphodiester SQRM appear to undergo significant hydrolysis after approx 45 min.

Chemical modifications to the internucleotide linkages would provide greater nuclease resistance of SQRMs *(4)*. In addition to modifications to the internucle-otide bridge, sugar or base alterations may also be expected to lend increased stability to these molecules *(5,6)*. More stabilized molecules could reasonably be expected to generate higher "signal-to-noise" ratios. Higher levels of fluores-cence might also be obtainable by redesigning loop sequence with impaired ability to undergo intramolecular folding. Alternatively, because mRNA-asso-ciated proteins and/or tertiary structure may govern the ability of SQRM to hybridize with their target, targeting different portions of the mRNA molecule might also be considered *(7,8)*. SQRM stabilization and higher signal-to-noise ratio would clearly be useful for more mechanistic studies on ODN sorting within cells and defining locations were duplex formation occurs most readily.

3. SQRM MAPPING OF MRNA

How one would rationally target SQRM to a particular mRNA species is still under investigation. More recently, we identified potential SQRM hybridization sites by a simple computer algorithm designed to locate complementary palin-dromic sequences approx 5–7 bases in length separated by intervening sequence (IVS) approx 18–20 nucleotides in length in the target RNA. Using this ap-proach, we scanned the mRNA sequences of a number of potential hematopoietic neoplasm gene targets including *c-myb*, c-*kit*, FLT3, STAT5, BCL2 and BCL6. Using the latter as an example, an insert containing full length BCL6 coding sequence was subcloned into pcDNA3 and then transcribed in vitro using T7 polymerase. Transcribed BCL6 RNA was introduced into wells on a 384 well plate, and individual SQRM, whose sequence was synthesized based on the target finding computer algorithm, were added to the wells in the presence of buffer containing 10 mM TRIS and 2 mM MgCl2. Fluorescence was quantitated over time in a plate reader and compared to an arbitrary 100% control, which was the exact DNA complement of the SQRM probe. Of 18 SQRM tested, one hybridized well yielding an approx 10-fold increase in fluorescence compared to background signal. To confirm hybridization with this probe, an in vitro RNase H-cleaving assay was carried out. Analysis on agarose gel demonstrated that the two expected fragments, approx 1.1kB and approx 1.3kB, respectively, could be visualized. "Hit" rates for the other targets was variable but ranged between 1 of 6 (*c-myb*) to 1 of 18 (BCL6). In the case of *c-myb* SQRM directed antisense oglionucleotide (asON) inhibited Myb protein expression approx 75% in living cells, without effect on β-actin protein. asON homologous to nonopening SQRM decreased Myb protein expression approx 20%. These results suggest that mRNA structure is an important consideration for NA-based RNA targeting, and that SQRM guided mapping can give highly relevant information useful for the design of more reliable NA probes and drugs.

4. CONCLUSIONS

A number of strategies for solving the problem of localizing mRNA sequence accessible for hybridization have been developed. These include trial-and-error ON "walks" 5' to 3' down the target mRNA sequence *(9)*, computer-assisted modeling of RNA structure *(10)*, hybridization of RNA to random ONs arrayed on glass slides *(11,12)*, and variations on the theme of using random ON libraries to identify RNase H cleavable sites, in the absence or presence of crude cellular extracts*(13–15)*. When employed in the context of the model, systems reported that these various methods are predictive, but their general applicability remains unclear. Furthermore, none offers the possibility of studying mRNA–probe interactions real time, in vitro, and, most importantly, in vivo. This is clearly an important consideration because the mRNA sequences of greatest, and most consistent, accessibility may only be revealed by in vivo probing of the cells of interest. Finally, this is the only technology that we are aware of that permits the study mRNA biology in real time, in living cells. Accordingly, we believe that the strategy outlined here represents an important advance in this field.

In addition to solving an important problem in the development of nucleic acid therapeutics, stabilized SQRM with strongly emitting fluorophore moieties may lend insight into the mechanism of action of antisense nucleic acids within cells. For example, when target mRNA is processed in the nucleus and exported to the cytoplasm, an SQRM duplexed with the mRNA should allow this transition to be monitored in real time by confocal fluorescence microscopy. If RNase H-assisted catalysis occurs in the nucleus, SQRM fluorescence would be lost in this location due to reformation of stem-loop sequences. The nuclei of effected cells would therefore appear dark. Alternatively, if RNase H-mediated degradation of the mRNA duplex does not occur, and the SQRM/mRNA hybrid is transported to the cytoplasm, it should be possible to demonstrate complex colocalization with ribosomes and possibly interference with translation if fluorescent signals remain in the same intracellular location. Other uses for the SQRM might easily be contemplated, including their use to study mRNA folding and processing, in vivo. SQRM might also act as reporters of viral invasion or the presence of mutated mRNA transcripts in vivo. With optimization of SQRM stability and fluorescence emission, these molecules will clearly become valuable tools for studying many aspects of RNA biology in living cells.

ACKNOWLEDGMENTS

Our work has been supported in part by NIH grants PO1 CA72765 and a grant from the Doris Duke Charitable Trust to AMG.

REFERENCES

1. Opalinska JB, Gewirtz AM. Nucleic-acid therapeutics: basic principles and recent applications. Nat Rev Drug Discov 2002; 1(7):503–514.
2. Tyagi S, Bratu SP, Kramer FR. Multicolor molecular beacons for allele discrimination. Nature Biotechnology 1998; 16:49–53.
3. Sokol DL, Zhang X, Gewirtz AM. Direct in vivo detection of hybridization between antisense oligodeoxynucleotides and target mRNA. Proc Natl Acad Sci USA 1998; 95:11,538–11,543.
4. Crooke ST. Advances in understanding the pharmacological properties of antisense oligonucleotides. Adv Pharmacol 1997; 40:1–49.
5. Lavignon M, et al. Inhibition of murine leukemia viruses by nuclease-resistant alpha-oligonucleotides. Antisense Res Dev 1992; 2(4):315–324.
6. Monia BP, et al. Evaluation of 2'-modified oligonucleotides containing 2'-deoxy gaps as antisense inhibitors of gene expression. J Biol Chem 1993; 268(19):14514–14522.
7. Gewirtz AM, Stein CA, Glazer PM. Facilitating oligonucleotide delivery: helping antisense deliver on its promise. Proc Natl Acad Sci USA 1996; 93(8):3161–3163.
8. Dewanjee MK, et al. Kinetics of hybridization of mRNA of c-myc oncogene with 111In-labeled antisense oligodeoxynucleotide probes by high-pressure liquid chromatography. Biotechniques 1994; 16(5):844–846, 848, 850.
9. Monia BP, et al. Sequence-specific antitumor activity of a phosphorothioate oligodeoxyribonucleotide targeted to human C-raf kinase supports an antisense mechanism of action in vivo. Proc Natl Acad Sci USA 1996; 93(26):15481–15484.
10. Sczakiel G, Homann M, Rittner K. Computer-aided search for effective antisense RNA target sequences of the human immunodeficiency virus type 1. Antisense Res Dev 1993; 3(1):45–52.
11. Milner N, Mir KU, Southern EM. Selecting effective antisense reagents on combinatorial oligonucleotide arrays [see comments]. Nat Biotechnol 1997; 15(6):537–541.
12. Sohail M, Southern EM. Selecting optimal antisense reagents. Adv Drug Deliv Rev 2000; 44(1):23–34.
13. Ho SP, et al. Mapping of RNA accessible sites for antisense experiments with oligonucleotide libraries [see comments]. Nat Biotechnol 1998; 16(1):59–63.

14. Scherr M, et al. RNA accessibility prediction: a theoretical approach is consistent with experimental studies in cell extracts. Nucleic Acids Res 2000; 28(13):2455–2461.

15. Ho SP, et al. RNA mapping: selection of potent oligonucleotide sequences for antisense experiments. Methods Enzymol 2000; 314:168–183.

V CLINICAL TARGETS

13 Nucleic Acids As Gene-Targeting Therapeutics

Joanna B. Opalinska, MD
and Susan E. Shetzline, PhD

1. INTRODUCTION

For diseases that are intrinsic to the human body, there is ultimately a molecular pathogenesis, either known or to be discovered. This being so, the possibility exists that manipulation of expression of the causative gene, or genes, could have significant therapeutic consequences. Furthermore, because biological processes are virtually always the result of the balance between stimulatory and inhibitory effects, it is difficult to imagine a situation where silencing a set of genes involved in one or the other of these effects couldn't be exploited for the purposes of treating disease. Such therapies might enjoy exquisite specificity, and in the case of malignant diseases in particular, might spare the patient from many morbid, and occasionally fatal, iatrogenic side effects. Hence the interest in molecular medicines.

From: *Cancer Drug Discovery and Development:*
Nucleic Acid Therapeutics in Cancer
Edited by: A. M. Gewirtz © Humana Press Inc., Totowa, NJ

Although conceptually elegant, a very large number of clinical trials, at least with antisense oligonucleotide (asON) drugs, have yet to prove the concept that gene-targeted therapies can favorably impact the course of a disease, or even to perform efficiently as gene-silencing agents *(1)*. The reasons for this are likely as complex as the biological systems in which they have been employed, but inefficient cellular delivery and lack of ability to designate hybridization accessible sequence within the targeted mRNA molecule are major stumbling blocks in this area. In this chapter we present a summary of the clinical experiences available for review in both malignant and nonmalignant diseases. More detailed discussions of specific targets may be found in the chapters following this one.

2. INHIBITION OF GENE EXPRESSION AS A TREATMENT FOR HEMATOLOGICAL MALIGNANCIES

Genetic rearrangements, mutations, and aberrant expression of genes have been associated with hematological malignancies. A classic example of a genetic rearrangement that has been directly linked to the pathogenesis of leukemia is the Philadelphia chromosome (Ph) translocation t(9;22) to generate the chimeric gene *BCR-ABL (2)*. Given that the constitutively elevated kinase activity of the Bcr-Abl fusion protein plays a critical role in its oncogenic potential and the exclusive expression of Bcr-Abl in chronic myelogenous leukemia (CML) cells, *BCR-ABL* is an attractive target for the treatment of CML. In fact, a number of ONs designed to silence *BCR-ABL* gene expression in CML cells have been utilized in vitro and ex vivo *(3–8)*. In vitro two *BCR-ABL* asOns, B3A2 and B2A2, have been used to determine their effect on cell growth. Only B3A2 inhibited K562 cell growth, which express Bcr-Abl, 44–63%, whereas both B3A2 and B2A2 inhibited peripheral blood stem/progenitor cell (PBSC) growth 124 and 98%, respectively *(8)*. In an independent study, *BCR-ABL* asONs directed against two *BCR-ABL* junctions suppressed leukemia colony formation, whereas granulocyte-macrophage colony formation from normal marrow progenitors remained unaffected *(7)*. Exposing a cell mixture of equal portions of normal marrow progenitors and blast cells to these *BCR-ABL* asONs ex vivo yielded residual colonies that were composed predominantly of normal cells, demonstrating that *BCR-ABL* is required for maintenance of a leukemic phentype. No significant toxicity was observed in the normal hematopoietic stem cell/progenitor cell population. The emergence of leukemia cells that are resistant to the small-molecule inhibitor Gleevec provides incentive to develop nucleic acid therapeutics instead of small-molecule inhibitors that proteins can easily evade through mutation.

Aberrant expression and mutated forms of *c-myb* have also been associated with hematological malignancies *(9–14)*. *c-Myb* is the normal homolog of the transforming avian myeloblastosis virus oncogene *v-myb (15–17)*. As a nuclear transcription factor expressed predominantly in hematopoietic cells *(18)*, *c-Myb* regulates the cell cycle at the G_1/S transition and plays a critical role in cell maturation *(19–21)*. When we exposed malignant hematopoietic cell lines and primary leukemia cells to *c-myb* antisense ODN, cell growth was inhibited *(22–26)*, indicating that *c-Myb* is also important for leukemic hematopoiesis. In view of the dramatic decrease in leukemic cell growth following treatment with *c-myb* asON, we hypothesized that *c-myb* asONs might serve as an effective therapeutic for leukemia. To test this hypothesis, we conducted clinical trials to evaluate the effectiveness of phosphorothioate modified *c-myb* asONs as marrow-purging agents for treating leukemia *(27)* and to determine the toxicity associated with intravenous infusion of these *c-myb* asONs into leukemia patients *(28)*. Our pilot marrow purging study consisted of Ph+ CML patients that were allograft ineligible. Following a 24-h ($n = 19$) or 72-h ($n = 5$) purge of the marrow with the *c-myb* asONs, a dramatic decline in *c-myb* mRNA levels was observed in approx 50% of the patients. Analysis of *BCR-ABL* gene expression in a surrogate stem-cell assay indicated that purging had been accomplished at a primitive cell level in >50% of the patients. Cytogenetics at day 100 in the surviving patients ($n = 14$) revealed two patients in complete cytogenetic remission, three patients with <33% Ph+ metaphases, and eight patients who remained 100% Ph+. Although the marrow of one patient yielded no metaphases, analysis of fluorescence *in situ* hybridization (FISH) results at approx 18 mo posttransplant revealed that approx 45% of cells expressed *BCR-ABL*, indicating that 6 out of 14 patients had originally obtained a "major" cytogenetic response. Our phase I systemic infusion study consisted of 18 refractory leukemia patients. Even though no recurrent dose-related toxicity was observed, two idiosyncratic toxicities were noted (one transient renal insufficiency; one pericarditis). One patient did survive for more than 14 mo with a transient restoration of chronic phase disease. The data from these studies demonstrate that *c-myb* asON may be administered safely to patients. The clinical benefit received by the patients in each study is uncertain. However, our initial observations suggest that antisense *c-myb* ON may serve as an effective therapy for hematological malignancies.

Overexpression of B-cell lymphoma protein 2 (BCL2), an *Myb*-regulated gene in hematopoietic cells that modulates apoptosis, has been implicated in the pathogenesis of some lymphomas like non-Hodgkin's lymphoma (NHL) *(29)*. Targeting BCL2 gene expression in the laboratory with asON specifically reduced BCL2 mRNA and protein levels six- to eightfold *(30)*. In a phase I clinical trial consisting of patients diagnosed with NHL, BCL2 expression was specifically decreased by sONs in 7 out of 16 patients *(31)*. This seemingly good inhibition of BCL2 expression in approx 50% of the study subjects did not correlate with obtaining a remission of the disease because only one patient had a complete response and two patients had minor responses to the asON. The absence of a direct correlation between tumor response and inhibition of BCL2 protein expression calls into question the mechanism by which the BCL2 asONs function to induce cell death.

Oligodeoxynucleotides (ODNs) have also been used as immunological adjuvants to treat NHL *(32)*. Unmethylated CpG motifs within bacterial ONs, or more germane to this discussion, synthetic ODNs are sufficient to illicit immune responses that have evolved to protect the host against infections. These immunological adjuvants have been postulated to function through a mechanism that involves the recognition of unmethylated CpG dinucleotides in certain base contexts (CpG) by pattern-recognition receptors on the surface of immune cells that can distinguish prokaryotic DNA from vertebrate DNA *(33)*. Responses of this type are similar to T-helper type 1 (T_H1)-cell responses, and lead to the activation of natural killer (NK) cells, dendritic cells, macrophages, and B cells *(34)*. In an independent study, CpG motifs within bacterial ODNs have been shown to directly activate B cells *(35)*. CpG DNA-induced immune activation has been shown to protect certain hosts against infection, either alone or in combination with vaccines. It is reasonable to suppose, then, that CpG-containing ODNs might prove to be effective adjuvants for the immunotherapy of cancer and for boosting immune responses to antigens that are less efficient in this regard, but to which one would like to immunize a host *(36)*. For these reasons, a clinical trial was conducted in which the safety and efficacy of a CpG adjuvant was investigated in 16 patients with NHL *(32)*. Analysis of the data indicated that the ODN increased the number and activity of NK cells in treated patients, and 2 out of 16 treated patients achieved partial remission. This study is continuing, and a follow-up clinical trial is planned in which study subjects will receive a combination of CpG ODNs with rituximab.

3. TARGETING GENE EXPRESSION AS A THERAPY FOR SOLID TUMOR CANCER

Nucleic acid drugs have also been utilized as a therapy for nonhematological malignancies. Gene targets have included protein kinase C (PKC)-α, which is discussed by Dr. Cho-Chung in Chapter 15, *h-ras*, C-*raf* kinase, *c-myb*, and BCL2. The transformation of many cell types has been attributed in part to a constitutively active RAS pathway and concomitant increase in proliferation. Based on these observations, a series of clinical trials were conducted using *h-ras* and C-*raf* asONs. In a phase I clinical trial, *h-ras* asONs were administered to patients with advanced cancer ($n = 23$) *(37)*. After receiving the nucleic acid drug for 14 d every 3 wk, only mild toxicities were observed. However, no complete or partial responses were achieved. Four patients had stabilized disease for 6 to 10 cycles of treatment. Since C-*raf* asONs have been shown to effectively inhibit the expression of its target gene in vitro *(38)* and in vivo tumor-xenograft model *(39)*, these ONs were used to determine their clinical efficacy *(40–42)*.

Seventy-eight patients were treated in these clinical trials. No major tumor responses were documented, but some patients had stabilization of their disease.

Aberrant expression of *Myb* and BCL2 has also been associated with nonhematological malignancies. Chromosome 6 rearrangement and alterations in *Myb* expression have been implicated in the pathogenesis of melanoma *(43–46)*. Exposing *Myb* positive human melanoma cells to unmodified or phosphoro-thioate-modified *c-myb* asONs inhibited cell growth in a dose- and sequence-dependent manner *(47)*. These in vitro assays also revealed that the inhibition of cell growth correlated with a specific decrease in the level of *c-myb* mRNA. Infusion of *c-myb* asON into severe combined immunodeficiency mice bearing human melanoma tumors transiently suppressed *c-myb* gene expression, but effected long-term growth suppression of transplanted tumor cells. Toxicity of the *c-myb* asON was minimal. Whereas *c-myb* antisense studies were conducted in a melanoma model, the *Myb*-regulated gene BCL2 was targeted by asONs for the treatment of patients with advanced malignant melanoma in combination with dacarbazine *(48)*. Of the 14 patients in this study, 1 had a complete response, 2 had a partial response, and 3 had a minor response. In an independent study, a combination therapy of BCL2 asON and mitoxantrone was used to treat patients ($n = 26$) with metastatic prostate cancer *(49)*. Only two patients had a decrease in the prostate-specific antigen. Studies with the BCL2 asON alone or in combination with chemotherapy agents have not shown consistent, strong antitumor responses. Understanding the mechanism of action of BCL2-based ONs might lead to the development of more effective nucleic acid therapeutics.

4. GENE-TARGETED THERAPEUTICS FOR NONMALIGNANT DISEASES

asONs have received attention as potential anti-inflammatory agents. A clinical example of postulated use in this regard is targeting the intracellular adhesion molecule-1 (ICAM-1) in Crohn's disease. The expression of ICAM-1 is elevated in many cells, but in this context is plays an important role in the migration and activation of leukocytes. It has been shown in vitro and in vivo that administration of ICAM-1 asONs causes a decrease in receptor expression, which in turn ameliorates inflammatory reactions *(50–52)*. Two clinical trials using this compound to treat patients with Crohn's disease have been reported *(53,54)*. In one double-blind study *(53)*, 20 patients were randomized to receive a saline placebo or anti-ICAM-asON. The treatment was well tolerated, and after 6 mo, disease remission was reported in 47% of patients in the antisense group compared with 20% of patients in the placebo group. Of interest, corticosteroid usage was significantly diminished ($p = 0.0001$) in the asON-treated patients. These results generated a great deal of excitement, but the enthusiasm was lessened by the follow-up study conducted on a larger cohort of patients ($n = 75$) *(54)*. In this placebo-controlled trial, no statistically significant differences in steroid use between the treatment or placebo groups was observed although "positive trends" were seen in the patients who were treated with the asON. As with other asON trials, toxicity was mild and consisted primarily of pain at the injection site, as well as fever and headache.

The anti-ICAM-1 ON has also been evaluated in patients with psoriasis. The compound was initially administered by intravenous infusion, but this mode of administration was abandoned when it was found that ON delivery to the various layers of skin was poor. Subsequently, a topical formulation was developed. Although preclinical data about uptake of this formulation into skin and down-regulation of expression of the gene target were again encouraging *(55)*, the ensuing clinical trial showed only modest, short-term effects in these patients. So as with other drugs of this class, the ultimate usefulness of this compound remains to be determined.

Cytokines released from cells in response to tissue injury that promote cell proliferation may also play a pivotal role in the pathogenesis of nonmalignant diseases. An example is the re-occlusion of coronary arteries that arises following angioplasty procedures performed on patients with atherosclerotic disease. Manipulation of coronary vessels invariably leads to endothelial cell injury, which is often accompanied by thrombosis, smooth muscle cell (SMC) activation, and subsequent vascular remodeling. Infusing antibodies against platelet-derived growth factor or basic fibroblast growth factor into SMCs have identified growth factors responsible for their proliferation and migration *(56)*. To identify and define the role of intracellular intermediates in these cellular processes, an asON approach appeared to be a logical strategy. The myelocytomatosis viral oncogene homolog *(c–myc)* has been identified as an important mediator in this process through its effects on regulating the growth of vascular cells in atherosclerotic lesions. Accordingly, it has been postulated that *c–myc* might make an attractive target for preventing postangioplasty complications, and at least two clinical trials using a 15-mer phosphorothioate-modified asON against *c–myc* have been reported *(57,58)*. Both studies demonstrated the safety of the nucleic acid drug in intracoronary applications, but no objective clinical responses were observed.

5. CONCLUSIONS

The use of reverse complementary nucleic acid drugs to inhibit gene expression originated from studies that were initiated almost a quarter of a century ago *(59,60)*. Although the mechanism by which these drugs modulate gene expression is not always clear *(61–63)*, the clinical development of nucleic acid drugs has proceeded to the point at which several of these drugs have entered phase I/II, and in a few cases, phase III trials. Results to date for most of these trials have been disappointing from the point of view of clinical efficacy. Nonetheless, the attraction for drugs of this class remains very strong, and has been revitalized the development of RNA interference *(64)*. This very exciting approach to gene silencing is, at the end of the day, also and "antisense-based methodology" whose robustness in a clinical setting also needs to be determined. Therefore, despite the fact that only one antisense nucleic acid drug has received Food and Drug Administration approval to date *(65)*, there is reason to remain optimistic that the problems that slow progress in this field will be overcome, and that many very useful drugs for the treatment of a variety of human and animal diseases will result.

REFERENCES

1. Opalinska JB, Gewirtz AM. Nucleic-acid therapeutics: basic principles and recent applications. Nat Rev Drug Discov 2002; 1(7):503–514.
2. Melo JV. The diversity of BCR-ABL fusion proteins and their relationship to leukemia phenotype. Blood 1996; 88(7):2375–2384.
3. Chasty R, Whetton A, Lucas G. A comparison of the effect of bcr/abl breakpoint specific phosphothiorate oligodeoxynucleotides on colony formation by bcr/abl positive and negative, CD34 enriched mononuclear cell populations. Leuk Res 1996; 20(5):391–395.
4. de Fabritiis P, Calabretta B. Antisense oligodeoxynucleotides for the treatment of chronic myelogenous leukemia: are they still a promise? Haematologica 1995; 80(4):295–299.
5. de Fabritiis P, Skorski T, De Propris MS, et al. Effect of bcr-abl oligodeoxynucleotides on the clonogenic growth of chronic myelogenous leukaemia cells. Leukemia 1997; 11(6):811–819.
6. Giles RV, Spiller DG, Green JA, Clark RE, Tidd DM. Optimization of antisense oligodeoxynucleotide structure for targeting bcr-abl mRNA. Blood 1995; 86(2):744–754.
7. Szczylik C, Skorski T, Nicolaides N, et al. Selective inhibition of leukemia cell proliferation by BCR-ABL antisense oligodeoxynucleotides. Science 1991; 253(5019):562–565.
8. Wu AG, Joshi SS, Chan WC, et al. Effects of BCR-ABL antisense oligonucleotides (AS-ODN) on human chronic myeloid leukemic cells: AS-ODN as effective purging agents. Leuk Lymphoma 1995; 20(1-2):67–76.
9. Barletta C, Pelicci PG, Kenyon LC, Smith SD, Dalla-Favera R. Relationship between the c-myb locus and the 6q-chromosomal aberration in leukemias and lymphomas. Science 1987; 235(4792):1064–1067.
10. Shetzline SE, Dowd KJ, Neely RJ, et al. A novel gene target of the c-Myb proto-oncogene in normal and malignant hematopoietic cells. Blood 2002; 100:742a.
11. Vorbrueggen G, Kalkbrenner F, Guehmann S, Moelling K. The carboxyterminus of human c-myb protein stimulates activated transcription in trans. Nucleic Acids Res 1994; 22(13):2466–2475.
12. Introna M, Golay J, Frampton J, Nakano T, Ness SA, Graf T. Mutations in v-myb alter the differentiation of myelomonocytic cells transformed by the oncogene. Cell 1990; 63(6):1289–1297.
13. Dini PW, Lipsick JS. Oncogenic truncation of the first repeat of c-Myb decreases DNA binding in vitro and in vivo. Mol Cell Biol 1993; 13(12):7334–7348.
14. Dini PW, Eltman JT, Lipsick JS. Mutations in the DNA-binding and transcriptional activation domains of v-Myb cooperate in transformation. J Virol 1995; 69(4):2515–2524.
15. Roussel M, Saule S, Langrow S, et al. Three types of viral oncogenes of cellular origin for haematopoietic cell transformation. Nature (London) 1979; 281:452–455.
16. Souza LM, Briskin MJ, Hillyard RL, Baluda MA. Identification of the avian myeloblastosis genome. J Virol 1980; 36:325–336.

17. Lipsick JS, Wang D-M. Transformation by v-Myb. Oncogene 1999; 18:3047–3055.
18. Kastan MB, Stone KD, Civin CI. Nuclear oncoprotein expression as a function of lineage, differentiation stage, and proliferative status of normal human hematopoietic cells. Blood 1989; 74(5):1517–1524.
19. Gewirtz AM, Calabretta B. A c-myb antisense oligodeoxynucleotide inhibits normal human hematopoiesis in vitro. Science 1988; 242(4883):1303–1306.
20. Caracciolo, D., D. Venturelli, M. Valtieri, C. Peschle, A.M. Gewirtz, and B. Calabretta, Stage-related proliferative activity determines c-myb functional requirements during normal human hematopoiesis. J Clin Invest, 1990. 85(1): p. 55–61.
21. Gewirtz AM, Anfossi G, Venturelli D, Valpreda S, Sims R, Calabretta B. G1/S transition in normal human T-lymphocytes requires the nuclear protein encoded by c-myb. Science 1989; 245(4914):180–183.
22. Anfossi G, Gewirtz AM, Calabretta B. An oligomer complementary to c-myb-encoded mRNA inhibits proliferation of human myeloid leukemia cell lines. Proc Natl Acad Sci USA 1989; 86(9):3379–3383.
23. Calabretta B, Sims RB, Valtieri M, et al. Normal and leukemic hematopoietic cells manifest differential sensitivity to inhibitory effects of c-myb antisense oligonucleotides: An in vitro study relevant to bone marrow purging. Proc Natl Acad Sci USA 1991; 88:2351–2355.
24. Ratajczak MZ, Hijiya N, Catani L, et al. Acute- and chronic-phase chronic myelogenous leukemia colony-forming units are highly sensitive to the growth inhibitory effects of c-myb antisense oligodeoxynucleotides. Blood 1992; 79(8):1956–1961.
25. Calabretta B, Gewirtz AM. Functional requirements of c-myb during normal and leukemic hematopoiesis. Crit Rev Oncog 1991; 2(3):187–194.
26. Ratajczak MZ, Kant JA, Luger SM, et al. In vivo treatment of human leukemia in a scid mouse model with c-myb antisense oligodeoxynucleotides. Proc Natl Acad Sci USA, 1992; 89(24):11823–11827.
27. Luger SM, O'Brien SG, Ratajczak J, et al. Oligodeoxynucleotide-mediated inhibition of c-myb gene expression in autografted bone marrow: a pilot study. Blood 2002; 99(4):1150–1158.
28. Gewirtz AM. Myb targeted therapeutics for the treatment of human malignancies. Oncogene 1999; 18:3056–3062.
29. Yang E, Korsmeyer SJ. Molecular thanatopsis: a discourse on the BCL2 family and cell death. Blood 1996; 88:386–401.
30. Reed JC, Stein C, Subasinghe C, et al., Antisense-mediated inhibition of BCL2 protooncogene expression and leukemic cell growth and survival: comparisons of phosphodiester and phosphorothioate oligodeoxynucleotides. Cancer Res 1990; 50(20):6565–6570.
31. Waters JS, Webb A, Cunningham D, et al. Phase I clinical and pharmacokinetic study of bcl-2 antisense oligonucleotide therapy in patients with non-Hodgkin's lymphoma. J Clin Oncol 2000; 18(9):1812–1823.
32. Jahrsdorfer B, Hartmann G, Racila E, et al. CpG DNA increases primary malignant B cell expression of costimulatory molecules and target antigens. J Leukoc Biol 2001; 69(1):81–88.
33. Krug A, Towarowski A, Britsch S, et al. Toll-like receptor expression reveals CpG DNA as a unique microbial stimulus for plasmacytoid dendritic cells which synergizes with CD40 ligand to induce high amounts of IL-12. Eur J Immunol 2001; 31(10):3026–3037.
34. Brazolot Millan CL, Weeratna R, Krieg AM, Siegrist CA, Davis HL. CpG DNA can induce strong Th1 humoral and cell-mediated immune responses against hepatitis B surface antigen in young mice. Proc Natl Acad Sci USA 1998; 95(26):15553–15558.
35. Krieg AM, Yi AK, Matson S, et al. CpG motifs in bacterial DNA trigger direct B-cell activation. Nature 1995; 374(6522):546–549.
36. Krieg AM, Yi AK, Schorr J, Davis and HL. The role of CpG dinucleotides in DNA vaccines. Trends Microbiol 1998; 6(1):23–27.

37. Cunningham CC, Holmlund JT, Geary RS, et al. A Phase I trial of H-ras antisense oligonucle-otide ISIS 2503 administered as a continuous intravenous infusion in patients with advanced carcinoma. Cancer 2001; 92(5):1265–1271.
38. Brennscheidt U, Riedel D, Kolch W, et al. Raf-1 is a necessary component of the mitogenic response of the human megakaryoblastic leukemia cell line MO7 to human stem cell factor, granulocyte-macrophage colony-stimulating factor, interleukin 3, and interleukin 9. Cell Growth & Differentiation 1994; 5(4):367–372.
39. Monia BP, Johnston JF, Geiger T, Muller M, Fabbro D. Antitumor activity of a phosphoro-thioate antisense oligodeoxynucleotide targeted against C-raf kinase. Nat Med 1996; 2(6):668–675.
40. Rudin CM, Holmlund J, Fleming GF, et al. Phase I Trial of ISIS 5132, an antisense oligonucle-otide inhibitor of c-raf-1, administered by 24-hour weekly infusion to patients with advanced cancer. Clin Cancer Res 2001; 7(5):1214–1220.
41. Cunningham CC, Holmlund JT, Schiller JH, et al. A phase I trial of c-Raf kinase antisense oligonucleotide ISIS 5132 administered as a continuous intravenous infusion in patients with advanced cancer. Clin Cancer Res 2000; 6(5):1626–1631.
42. Coudert B, Anthoney A, Fiedler W, et al. Phase II trial with ISIS 5132 in patients with small-cell (SCLC) and non-small cell (NSCLC) lung cancer. A European Organization for Research and Treatment of Cancer (EORTC) Early Clinical Studies Group report. Eur J Cancer 2001; 37(17):2194–2198.
43. Linnenbach AJ, Huebner K, Reddy EP, et al. Structural alteration in the MYB protooncogene and deletion within the gene encoding alpha-type protein kinase C in human melanoma cell lines. Proc Natl Acad Sci USA 1988; 85(1):74–78.
44. Trent JM, Thompson FH, Meyskens FLJ. Identification of a recurring translocation site in-volving chromosome 6 in human malignant melanoma. Cancer Res 1989; 49(2):420–423.
45. Meese E, Meltzer PS, Witkowski CM, Trent JM. Molecular mapping of the oncogene MYB and rearrangements in malignant melanoma. Genes Chromosomes Cancer 1989; 1(1):88–94.
46. Dasgupta P, Linnenbach AJ, Giaccia AJ, Stamato TD, Reddy EP. Molecular cloning of the breakpoint region on chromosome 6 in cutaneous malignant melanoma: evidence for deletion in the c-myb locus and translocation of a segment of chromosome 12. Oncogene 1989; 4(10):2101–2105.
47. Hijiya N, Zhang J, Ratajczak MZ, et al. Biologic and therapeutic significance of MYB expres-sion in human melanoma. Proc Natl Acad Sci USA 1994; 91(10):4499–4503.
48. Jansen B, Wacheck V, Heere-Ress E, et al. Chemosensitisation of malignant melanoma by BCL2 antisense therapy. Lancet 2000; 356(9243):1728–1733.
49. Chi KN, Gleave ME, Klasa R, et al. A phase I dose-finding study of combined treatment with an antisense Bcl-2 oligonucleotide (Genasense) and mitoxantrone in patients with metastatic hormone-refractory prostate cancer. Clin Cancer Res 2001; 7(12):3920–3927.
50. Bennett CF, Condon TP, Grimm S, Chan H, Chiang MY. Inhibition of endothelial cell adhesion molecule expression with antisense oligonucleotides. J Immunol 1994; 152(7):3530–3540.
51. Nestle FO, Mitra RS, Bennett CF, Chan H, Nickoloff BJ. Cationic lipid is not required for uptake and selective inhibitory activity of ICAM-1 phosphorothioate antisense oligonucle-otides in keratinocytes. J Invest Dermatol 1994; 103(4):569–575.
52. Miele ME, Bennett CF, Miller BE, Welch DR. Enhanced metastatic ability of TNF-alpha-treated malignant melanoma cells is reduced by intercellular adhesion molecule-1 (ICAM-1, CD54) antisense oligonucleotides. Exp Cell Res 1994; 214(1):231–241.
53. Yacyshyn BR, Bowen-Yacyshyn MB, Jewell L, et al. A placebo-controlled trial of ICAM-1 antisense oligonucleotide in the treatment of Crohn's disease. Gastroenterology 1998; 114(6):1133–1142.

54. Schreiber S, Nikolaus S, Malchow H, et al. Absence of efficacy of subcutaneous antisense ICAM-1 treatment of chronic active Crohn's disease. Gastroenterology 2001; 120(6):1339–1346.

55. Wraight CJ, White PJ, McKean SC, et al. Reversal of epidermal hyperproliferation in psoriasis by insulin-like growth factor I receptor antisense oligonucleotides. Nat Biotechnol 2000; 18(5):521–526.

56. Rosenberg, RD. Vascular smooth muscle cell proliferation: basic investigations and new therapeutic approaches. Thromb Haemost 1993; 70(1):10–16.

57. Roque F, Mon G, Belardi J, et al. Safety of intracoronary administration of c-myc antisense oligomers after percutaneous transluminal coronary angioplasty (PTCA). Antisense Nucleic Acid Dev 2001; 11(2):99–106.

58. Kutryk MJ, Foley DP, van den Brand M, et al. Local intracoronary administration of antisense oligonucleotide against c-myc for the prevention of in-stent restenosis: results of the randomized investigation by the Thoraxcenter of antisense DNA using local delivery and IVUS after coronary stenting (ITALICS) trial. J Am Coll Cardiol 2002; 39(2):281–287.

59. Paterson BM, Roberts BE, Kuff EL. Structural gene identification and mapping by DNA-mRNA hybrid-arrested cell-free translation. Proc Natl Acad Sci USA 1977; 74(10):4370–4374.

60. Stephenson ML, Zamecnik PC. Inhibition of Rous sarcoma viral RNA translation by a specific oligodeoxyribonucleotide. Proc Natl Acad Sci USA 1978; 75(1):285–288.

61. Gewirtz AM. Oligonucleotide therapeutics: a step forward. J Clin Oncol 2000; 18:1809–1811.

62. Scherr M, Rossi JJ, Sczakiel G, Patzel V. RNA accessibility prediction: a theoretical approach is consistent with experimental studies in cell extracts. Nucleic Acids Res 2000; 28:2455–2461.

63. Stein CA. Does antisense exist? Nat Med 1995; 1:1119–1121.

64. Shuey DJ, McCallus DE, Giordano T. RNAi: gene-silencing in therapeutic intervention. Drug Discov Today 2002; 7(20):1040–1046.

65. De Smet MD, Meenken C, van den Horn GJ. Fomivirsen-a phosphorothioate oligonucleotide for the treatment of CMV retinitis. Ocul Immunol Inflamm 1999; 7:189–198.

14   Y900003 (Isis 3521) and G3139 (Genasense; Oblimersen)

Phosphorothioate Antisense Oligonucleotides With Pleiotropic Mechanisms of Action

C. A. Stein, MD, PhD, Nathalie Dias, PhD, Luba Benimetskaya, PhD, Jan S. Jepsen, BS, Johnathan C. H. Lai, BS, and Anthony J. Raffo, PhD

"The thing is not done well, but it is remarkable that it is done at all."

Dr. Samuel Johnson, referring to a dancing dog, as quoted by James Boswell, *Life of Johnson*

The chemical synthesis of stereorandom phosphorothioate oligodeoxynucleotides (ODN) was first performed in 1984 by Wojciech Stec and his colleagues

From: *Cancer Drug Discovery and Development:*
Nucleic Acid Therapeutics in Cancer
Edited by: A. M. Gewirtz © Humana Press Inc., Totowa, NJ

(1,2). Ever since, these molecules have essentially formed one of the most important elements of antisense oligonucleotide (asON) biotechnology. Several of these constructs have relatively recently entered phase II and even phase III clinical therapeutic trials for cancer indications, with encouraging preliminary results *(3–5)*. In fact, the single Food and Drug Administrationapproved asON drug, Vitravene (for cytomegalovirus retinitis), is a phosphorothioate ODN.

The relative longevity of phosphorothioate ODNs appears all the more remarkable given that their scientific "obituary" has been written many times over a very long period of time. However, the fact that they are still of such intense interest is a telling comment on their remarkable biological activity *(6,7)*. The purpose of this chapter is to dissect this activity, and to demonstrate that it depends on a complex mixture of mechanisms, some related to antisense effects, others not.

1. BASIC BIOLOGIC PROPERTIES OF PHOSPHOROTHIOATE ODNS

Phosphorothioate ODNs, which contain a sulfur atom substituted for an oxygen atom at a nonbridging site at each phosphorus in the ON chain (Fig. 1), were originally prepared to vitiate the problem of nuclease digestion in biological systems, which is predominately the result of the ubiquitous presence of 3' exonuclease activity *(8,9)*. This substitution retains the negative charge of the ON, and hence the critical property of aqueous solubility. However, although stereorandom phosphorothioates hybridize to targeted, complementary mRNA sequences, the values of Tm (melting temperature) are significantly lower than that of the isosequential phosphodiester ON (about 1.5°C lower for each GC pair and about 0.5°C lower for each AT pair) *(10)*.

Although the phosphorothioate substitution does render ONs nuclease resistant, it by no means makes them nuclease proof. Actually, phosphorothioates are degraded both intracellularly and in vivo (particularly in the plasma, kidney, and liver) *(8,9)*, a fact that may be of some significance if the degradation products have intrinsic biological activity. This is especially likely in the in vivo setting, owing to the observation that, in contrast to what has been observed in experiments in tissue culture, it does not seem that carriers need to be employed in order to produce antisense effects. A dramatic, and perhaps the finest, demonstration of this principle was recently provided by Zhang et al. *(11)*, who, in well-controlled experiments, targeted the hepatic expression of *fas* in the liver of Balb/c mice. Not only was the hepatocyte cell-surface expression of *fas* down-regulated, but the lethality of an anti-*fas* monoclonal antibody was completely blocked. However, questions and rumors have recently arisen about the reproducibility of these data, although nothing that definitively addresses this important proof of principle has been published. Furthermore, it must still be considered

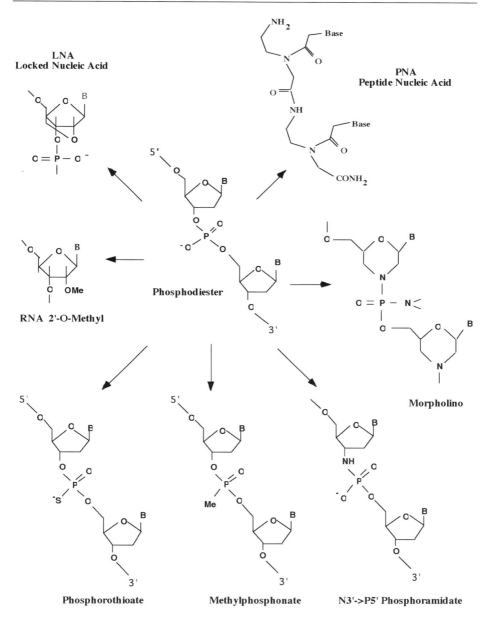

Fig. 1. Different chemical modifications of oligonucleotides.

uncertain that such effects can be produced in other organs whose uptake of ONs can only modestly approach that of the liver.

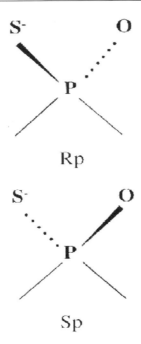

Fig. 2. Stereochemical representation of the Rp and Sp phosphorus atom in a phosphorothioate linkage.

That phosphorothioate ON degradation products can affect cellular pheno-types no longer seems in doubt; witness the results of Koziolkiewicz et al. *(8)*, who demonstrated that treatment of HL60 cells with 5'-deoxynucleoside monothiophosphates may variably affect cellular proliferation. Sometimes, in fact, as in the case of deoxyguanylic acid, the proliferation rate may actually be increased by approx 50%. (Other nucleotide monophosphorothioates [NMPS], depending on the cell line treated, can decrease proliferation to approximately the same extent.) Furthermore, it is also clear that the $n - 1$, $n - 2$, etc. 3'-degradation products of an antisense phosphorothioate ON are not entirely inac-tive and may also act as antisense agents, although perhaps, at least in some cases, via a somewhat different mechanism than what had been observed for the paren-tal molecule *(12)*. These observations will be further discussed later.

Phosphorothioates possess a sense of chirality, occurring as Rp and Sp diaste-reomers, which, by definition, are mirror images of each other (Fig. 2). The Sp diastereomer, however, is inherently helix destabilizing, as it points "in" to the major groove of the double helix formed by hybridization between a phosphoro-thioate ON and RNA. The Rp stereoisomer points "out," and hence does not steri-cally destabilize the double helix *(13,14)*. However, the Rp stereoisomer is relatively nuclease sensitive and may be degraded by nucleases almost as rapidly by 3'-exonuclease activity as the isosequential phosphodiester ON *(15,16)*. On the other hand, the Sp ON is highly nuclease-resistant, and it has been demonstrated that even a single Sp linkage at the 3' terminus of a phosphorothioate ON can protect it against nuclease digestion *(16)*. The incorporation of such a linkage would therefore block the release of deoxyribonucleoside monophosphates, and prevent their toxic or stimulatory effects on cell growth. Furthermore, the use of stereoregular phosphorothioate linkages to block 3' nuclease digestion eliminates the need for nonnucleotide 3' protecting groups and provides for the most minimal possible modification of the structure or backbone of the asON. This, at least in theory, would provide a more biochemically coherent way of assessing to what extent the phenotype obtained from a given experiment was truly due to the down-regulation of the target, or whether the phenotype was in fact mostly the result of effects of the degradation products of the parental oligomer. (As discussed later, the non-antisense effects of the parental phosphorothioate ON may contribute significantly to the observed phenotype in an antisense experiment.) However, such 3' stereoregular ONs cannot be obtained commercially and at the present time can only be obtained in small quantities from a very limited number of sources *(1,17–19)*.

2. NONSEQUENCE-SPECIFIC EFFECTS OF PHOSPHOROTHIOATE ONS

Phosphorothioate ON are polyanions and as such bind to the same molecules as naturally occurring polyanions (e.g., heparin, heparan sulfate) *(20,21)*. Phosphodiester ONs will also bind to heparin-binding molecules, but do so with affinities approximately one to three orders of magnitude lower than the isosequential phosphorothioate ON. There are many examples of heparin-binding proteins in the literature that can be bound with high affinity and, in a length-dependent fashion, by phosphoro-thioates. For example, basic fibroblast growth factor *(21)* has been shown to bind to SdC28 with $Kd = 3$ nM (Fig. 3), and the growth factor is removed by this oligomer from its low-affinity binding sites on bovine corneal endothelial matrix. Many other phosphorothioate ONs of the same length behave similarly. Other heparin-binding growth factors, such as platelet-derived growth factor and vascular endothelial growth factor (VEGF), as well as receptors for VEGF, can also bind to phosphorothioate ONs *(22)*. Epidermal growth factor (EGF) (in contrast to the EGF receptor [EGFR]) is not heparin-binding and does not bind to phosphorothioates. However, SdC28 does interact with EGFR, and blocks its phosphorylation in the presence of EGF by preventing the receptor–ligand interaction. Interestingly, in the absence of EGF, SdC28 promotes auto-phosphorylation of EGFR *(22)*. Phosphorothioates can also, at relatively high concentration, block cellular adhesion to artificial surfaces by interacting with fibronectin and laminin *(23)* and preventing their nor-

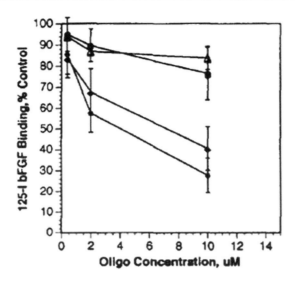

Fig. 3. Inhibition of basic growth factor binding to NIH 3T3 cells by phosphorothioate and phosphodiester homopolymers. 10^6 NIH 3T3 cells per well were plated in six-well plates to obtain the desired full confluence on the next day. Before the initiation of the binding reaction, cells were washed twice with Dulbecco's phosphate-buffered saline (DPBS) and incubated for 1 h in medium with 0.1% (w/v) bovine serum albumin (BSA) at 37°C. The binding reactions were all achieved at 4°C. Cells were incubated in serum-free medium containing 0.1% BSA, 0.05 mg/mL ^{125}I-basic fibroblast growth factor (bFGF), and 0.5, 2, and 10 μM of the desired phosphorothioate (S) and phosphodiester (O) oligonucleotides (●, SdC28; ◆, SdT28; ■, OdC25; Δ, OdT25). After 2 h, medium was removed, and cell-bound bFGF was measured after washing three times the cells with DPBS and lysing them with 1M NaOH. The amount of radioactivity was measured by γ counting.

mal functioning, including, in the case of laminin, blocking the binding of it to sulfatide, its natural ligand. These ONs may also have an antimetastatic function as, similar to other classes of polyanion such as suramin *(24)* and polysulfated polysaccharides *(25)*, they nonspecifically interfere with heparanase, the major β-1,4-endoglycosidase in mammalian metastatic tumor deposits *(25)*. However, unlike suramin (and similar to polysulfated polysaccharides), phosphorothioate oligonucleotides do not interact with adenosine 5'-triphosphate-binding sites *(26)*. All of these effects, incidentally, appear to be independent of the sense of chirality at phosphorus *(27)*.

Gao et al. *(28)* were perhaps the first to appreciate that phosphorothioate ONs could also bind nonspecifically to RNase H. This, of course, means that this class of oligomer may in fact nonspecifically inhibit the very class of enzyme that is most responsible for the antisense effect. However, to what extent this mechanism actually contributes to lack of antisense efficacy either in vitro or in vivo remains unclear. In addition to the downregulation of the activity of large numbers of proteins, only some of which have been mentioned here, phosphorothioate ONs also appear to stimulate the activity of the Sp1 transcription factor *(29)*. This effect appears to be independent of length and sequence. The specific consequences of such activation of a critical transcription factor have not yet been fully elucidated.

Because of the intrinsic problem of nonspecific toxicity of phosphorothioate ONs owing to their polyanionic character, several attempts have been made to define appropriate controls when antisense experiments using these molecules are performed *(7,30)*. Suffice to say that at this point this remains a controversial area, and one that is not likely to be entirely resolved any time soon. But it is also true that the question of appropriate controls is of diminished importance when phosphorothioate ONs are employed for therapeutic purposes vs for the validation of gene function. In the former, issues of efficacy vs toxicity almost invariably trump mechanistic questions; in the latter, mechanistic problems become paramount, especially when they impact on the appropriate interpretation of experimental data. In fact, it is our contention that true sequence specificity does not exist for phosphorothioate ONs. Alternatively phrased, we do not believe it is possible to extrapolate backward from a phenotype to a specific target knockout when phosphorothioates are employed. In other words, the claim that a particular protein (whose expression has been down-regulated in the experiments) is responsible for a specific phenotype is not tenable. However, it may be possible to extrapolate in the reverse, negative, sense. For example, if a protein is proposed to be anti-apoptotic, and the downregulation of its expression by a phosphorothioate ON does not lead to cellular apoptosis, then it is likely that the protein in question is probably not a good anti-apoptotic target. This is an important distinction, especially when a high-throughput method for negatively validating large numbers of targets is required.

3. RNASE H-INDUCED CLEAVAGE OF NONTARGETED MRNAS

Based on charge considerations, the longer a phosphorothioate oligomer is, the more nonspecific it becomes *(21,31,32)*. However, the presence of increasing numbers of phosphorothioate linkages is not the only reason for increasing ON "nonspecificity" as a function of length *(33)*. In fact, paradoxically, nonspecificity also increases as a function of increasing base content, irrespective of backbone (provided the backbone is charged) *(34,35)*. This is the result of the properties of RNase H, the enzyme that cleaves the mRNA strand at the point of hybridization to complementary DNA *(36,37)*. It was first noted by Cazenave et al. *(38)* that RNase H in wheatgerm extract could cleave the mRNA of β-globin if only 13 bp of a 17-mer ON were complementary to it. Furthermore, Monia et al. *(39)* determined that even very short regions of complementarity (perhaps 5- or even 4-

mer) could, under some circumstances, be sufficient to be recognized by RNase H. This plays out in a very interesting way, as Giles and Tidd *(34,35)* have described. In their analysis, any 15-mer can be viewed as 8 overlapping 8-mers. However, the occurrence of each 8-mer, with its RNase H cleavage sites, would be expected to occur about once in every 6.55 (10^4 bases of random mRNA sequence. Considerations of sequence homology, would predict an occurrence of only 1 in 10^9, however, which is far more infrequent than 1 in 6.55 ° 10^4 (or 1 in 8192 for the sum of the 8). However, it is quite likely, given the extensive self-hybridization of mRNA and the relatively strict requirements *(40)* for the formation of DNA–RNA duplexes, that many of the 1 in 8192 sites are not available for ON binding.

Regardless, the ability of RNase H to cleave nontargeted mRNA species is most likely dependent not only on oligomer length but also oligomer concentration and binding affinity to targeted mRNA decreases with increasing mismatches. Intracellular ON concentration, in turn, depends on the external ON concentration, but, more important perhaps, on the nature of the delivery vehicle (e.g., cationic lipid, polyamine, peptide). For example, in T24 bladder carcinoma cells, Isis 3521 (a.k.a. LY900003), a 20-mer phosphorothioate oligomer targeted to the 3'-UTR of the protein kinase C (PKC)-α mRNA, down-regulates PKC-α protein and mRNA expression, but not PKC-β1 and ζ, when delivered by lipofectin *(41,42)*. On the other hand, when delivered by the cationic porphyrin meso tetra(methylpyridyl)porphine, both PKC-α and -ζ (but not PKC-β1, δ or ε) protein expression were down-regulated *(43)* (Fig. 4). In addition, the levels of the 4.0 and 2.2 kb PKC-ζ mRNA transcripts were reduced by about 95%. Because there is a contiguous 11-bases match between Isis 3521 and the PKC-ζ mRNA, which is more than sufficient for recognition by RNase H, it is likely that the down-regulation of PKC-ζ mRNA and protein activity is the result of the cleavage of a nontargeted mRNA *(43)*.

As follows from this discussion, a reduction in the cleavage of nontargeted mRNAs would be important if it is important to determine the precise relationship between an antisense knockout and a cellular phenotype. (Whether such a reduction would be beneficial or, in fact, deleterious in the therapeutic setting is currently unclear). RNase H requires an ON to be charged in order for it to recognize a potentially cleavable duplex (although not all charged ONs are RNase H competent) *(39,44–46)*. The enzyme also requires one strand to be composed of at least some contiguous deoxyribonucleotide linkages. This means that ONs composed solely of methylphosphonate, or 2'-*O*-alkyl (e.g., *O*-methyl or *O*-methoxyethoxy) oligoribonucleotide linkages are not RNase H competent *(39,46)*. Indeed, these linkages have been incorporated into ONs to reduce RNase H competency (and increase target affinity) and hence the cleavage of nontargeted mRNAs *(34,39,45,47)*. (Because of nuclease sensitivity, the phosphorothioate backbone is retained in a 2'-*O*-alkyl ON). However, ONs that cannot elicit RNase H activity lose their "pseudo-catalytic" activity and thus tend to be inefficient antisense

-24 ————————————————TGA-A-AC—T-CACCAGCGAG— 25
1601 CAGACGACTACGGTCTGGACAACTTTGACACACAGTTCACCAGCGAGCCC
1650

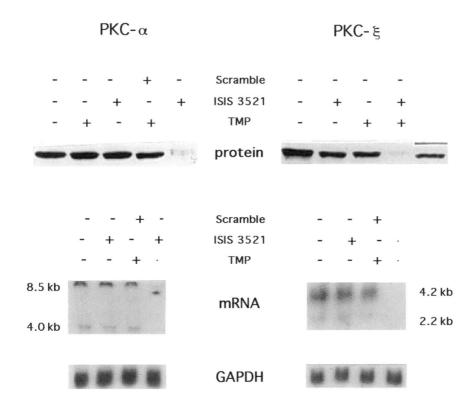

Fig. 4. Downregulation of PKC isoform proteins in T24 bladder cancer cells by phosphorothioate oligonucleotides.Twenty-five 10^4 T24 cells per well were seeded in six-well plates to be 70 to 80% confluent on the next day. Cells were treated for 5 h with preformed complexes of porphyrin (TMP) (9 μM) and oligonucleotides (3 μM). Cells were washed with complete medium and then, after 19 h, harvested and lysed in 50 mM Tris-HCl, pH 7.4, 1% Nonidet P-40, 0.25% sodium deoxycholate, 150 mM NaCl, 1 mM EGTA, 1 mM Na$_3$VO$_4$, 1 mM NaF, 1 mM PMSF and 1 mg/mL aprotinin and leupeptin. For Western blot analysis, 25–40 μg of proteins were resolved into a 10% sodium dodecyl sulfate polyacrylamide gel and then blotted to Hybond ECL membrane. The membrane was probed first with the anti-protein kinase C (PKC) isoform-specific antibodies and then with the peroxidase-conjugated secondary antibody. The revelation was performed with ECL. For Northern blot analysis, total RNA was isolated with TRIZOL Reagent. 20–30 μg of total RNA was resolved into a 1.2% agarose-formaldehyde gel and transferred to a Hybond-N nylon membrane. The membrane was probed with a random-primed (32) P-radiolabeled cDNA probes corresponding to the human PKC-α and PKC-ξ or the human glyceraldehyde-3-phosphate dehydrogenase (GAPDH). Them membrane was then exposed to a Kodak X-ray film and quantified.

effector molecules *(48,49)*, perhaps because of the unwinding activity of the 80S ribosome *(50)*. Such RNase H-incompetent molecules are in fact only active when targeted at relatively high concentration to the 5'-UTR of the mRNA *(51,52)*. (Some RNase H-incompetent ONs, such as peptide nucleic acids, have very high Tms, but are poorly soluble and hence difficult to deliver into the cell nucleus *(48,53)*. Others, such as N3'-P5' phosphoramidates, tend to produce nonsequence-specific effects. Locked-nucleic acids appear to have an even higher affinity for RNA than do the peptide nucleic acids *(54,55)* and, even when only a few are incorporated into each phosphorothioate ON, will also undoubtedly produce significant nonsequence specificity (Jepsen and Stein, personal observation).

At the present time, suppression of the cleavage of nontargeted mRNA species is probably best accomplished by the "gap-mer" strategy. Four or more 2'-*O*-alkyl oligoribonucleotide linkages are incorporated into the 3' and 5' termini of the oligomer, whereas the central region (at least 6 bases) remains oligodeoxyribonucleotide phosphorothioate in order to preserve RNase H activity *(56,57)*. However, the gap-mer strategy by no means eliminates all cleavage of nontargeted mRNAs *(58)*. Indeed, its very effectiveness at diminishing the cleavage of nontargeted mRNAs can be vitiated if the backbone has been modified to increase the affinity of the oligonucleotide for its mRNA target *(59)*.

To eliminate the problem of the cleavage of nontargeted mRNAs and the nonspecific effects of phosphorothioates, we *(60)* and others *(61–63)*, have developed an RNase H-independent strategy to produce specific target inhibition, which instead depends on mRNA cleavage by RNase P. The function of this ubiquitous ribozyme-containing protein is to cleave the leader 5' terminus of precursor transfer RNA (tRNA) to generate a mature tRNA *(64)*. ONs of the appropriate length that mimic certain structural features of the precursor tRNA can be recognized intracellularly by RNase P, leading to mRNA cleavage and down-regulation of protein and mRNA expression (Fig. 5). These ONs lack phosphorothioate in the backbone and have had their 3' termini stabilized by a 3'-3' inverted thymidine residue. Such RNase P-competent ONs have been used to treat several bladder cancer cell lines, and specific down-regulation of both PKC-α and bcl-xL protein, and mRNA expression has been demonstrated *(60)*.

4. LY900003 (ISIS 3521) AND G3139 (GENASENSE; OBLIMERSEN): PHOSPHOROTHIOATE ANTISENSE OLIGONUCLEOTIDES WITH PLEOTROPIC MECHANISMS OF ACTION

In high passage number PC3 prostate cancer cells, both Isis 3521 and G3139 appear to sensitize cells to the cytotoxic effects of paclitaxel *(12)* (Fig. 6). In our initial experiments with Isis 3521, we wanted to determine how 3'-base truncation mutants and 3' protection by a single Sp phosphorothioate linkage affected

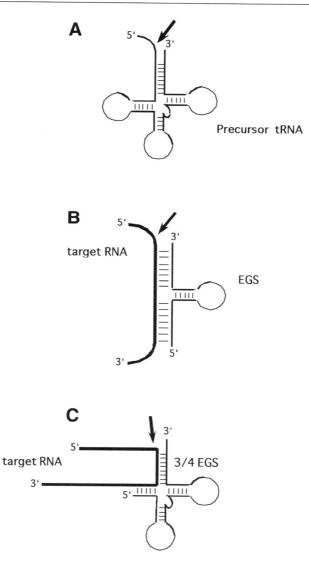

Fig. 5. Model substrates for ribonuclease P (RNase P). (**A**) Structure of a precursor tRNA. (**B** and **C**) Representation of tRNA-like EGS structures. EGS hybridize to the targeted RNA through Watson–Crick basepairing and form a structure that resemble to the tRNA. The arrow represents the site of natural cleavage by RNase P. (**C** is from ref. *64.*)

this sensitivity. Surprisingly, all ONs, down to a 13-mer in length, were identical with respect to their ability to down-regulate the expression of PKC-α protein (approx 82 +/– 2% downregulation, as assessed by laser scanning densitometry

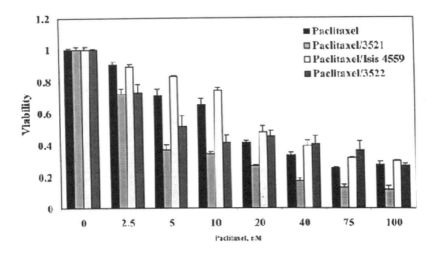

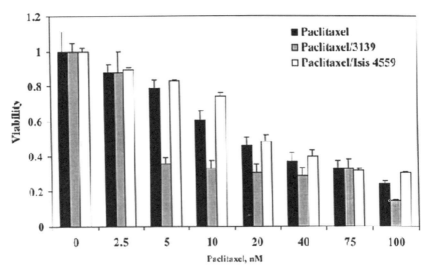

Fig. 6. Chemosensitization of T24 bladder cancer cells to paclitaxel after treatment with the phosphorothioate anti-Bcl2 G3139 or anti-PKC-α ISIS 3521 oligonucleotides. 0.6–1 10⁴ T24 cells per well were seeded in 96-well microtiter plates. Cells were treated during 5 h with preformed complexes of lipofectin (10 μg/mL) and the anti-Bcl-2 G3139 or anti-PKC-α ISIS3521 oligonucleotides (1 μ*M*). After the oligonucleotide treatment, various concentrations of paclitaxel were added to the medium and the cell viability was tested with a MTT assay after 3 d of incubation. Absorbance was determined at 540 nm with a MR600 microplate reader and the values were normalized to the controls.

of the Western blots). Furthermore, the rate at which PKC-α protein expression decreased, and then reappeared within several days after ON treatment, was identical for all the ONs. However, the response to treatment of PKC-α mRNA expression did not necessarily correlate with the protein response. Treatment of the cells with 16-mer and longer oligonucleotides led to a sharp decrease in PKC-α mRNA levels. However, treatment of the cells with a 15-mer or shorter molecules did not lead to any decrease in the expression of PKC-α mRNA, despite the fact that levels of protein expression were down-regulated to the same extent for both the 15-mer and the 20-mer. This appears to indicate that the down-regulation of PKC-α protein expression occurs by two distinct mechanisms: one RNase H dependent at longer ON length; and the other, RNase H independent. The origin of the RNase H-independent mechanism is currently uncertain, and is currently a subject of great interest to us.

To improve intracellular ON stability, we, in collaboration with Wojciech Stec and Serge Beaucage and their respective groups, evaluated PKC-α 3'-truncation mutations (17-, 16-, and 15-mers) containing 3'-terminal single Sp linkages *(12)*. As mentioned previously, the Sp, as opposed to the Rp diastereomer, is highly nuclease resistant. For both the 17-mer and the 16-mer, the terminal Sp diastereomer produced a significantly more chemosensitizing ON vs the parental 3' Sp/Rp diastereomeric mixture (Fig. 7). However, for the 15-mer, very little increase in sensitivity to paclitaxel, vs treatment with paclitaxel alone, was observed, despite the fact that PKC-α protein expression was down-regulated to the same extent in all cases. We conclude, in this case, that down-regulation of PKC-α expression may be necessary but is not sufficient to generate chemosensitivity. Therefore, it is possible that all the other biological activities of Isis 3521, for example, the nonspecific binding to proteins, the ability to elicit RNase H cleavage of nontargeted mRNAs, and, in addition, other hitherto unknown properties are acting in combination with the down-regulation of PKC-α protein expression to induce chemosensitivity. The ON length-dependent decrease in chemosensitization is consistent with this idea, as the shorter the oligomer, the less nonspecific it is, and the more reduced its ability to support the cleavage of nontargeted mRNAs by RNase H. However, the hypothesis that PKC-α protein expression is just a marker for other, perhaps unrelated, events is also consistent with these data.

To our surprise, we somewhat serendipitously found that G3139, in addition to downregulating bcl-2 protein and mRNA expression, also downregulated the expression of PKC-α protein and mRNA, but not the expression of other PKC isoforms (Fig. 8). Furthermore, we were able to separate out the effects on chemosensitivity of bcl-2 down-regulation from PKC-α down-regulation by using a lipid mixture called Eufectin 5 (no longer commercially available) as the ON carrier *(12)*. In T24 bladder carcinoma cells, at a 50-n*M* concentration of G3139 in complex with Eufectin 5, only bcl-2 expression was down-regulation (Fig. 9). At a 100-n*M* concentration, both PKC-α and bcl-2 expression were

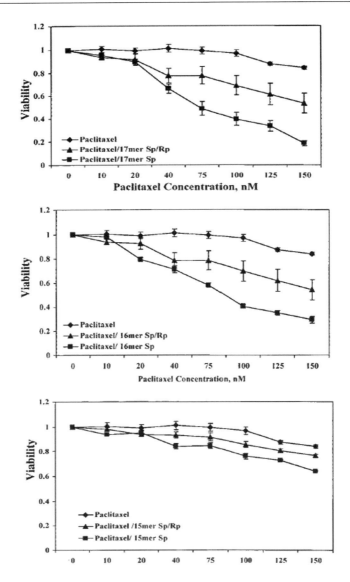

Fig. 7. Effect of the chirality of the terminal phosphorothioate on chemosensitization of T24 cells to paclitaxel. Truncated phosphorothioate oligonucleotides (17-, 16-, and 15-mer), with 3'-Sp-diastereoisomer and parental 3'-Sp/Rp mixture, were tested in cell viability assays. T24 cells were harvested in 96-well microtiter plates and were treated 5 h the next day with 3'-truncated oligonucleotides (1 μM), previously complexed to lipofectin (10 µg/mL). After 3 d of incubation with various concentrations of paclitaxel, cell viability was measured by MTT assay. Absorbance at 540 nm was normalized to the control untreated cells.

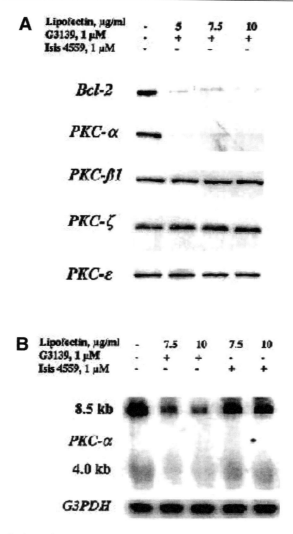

Fig. 8. Downregulation of Bcl-2 and PKC-α proteins by the antisense phosphorothioate G3139 oligonucleotide in T24 bladder cancer cells. Twenty 10^4 T24 cells per well were seeded in six-well plates to be 70 to 80% confluent on the next day. Cells were treated for 5 h with preformed complexes of various concentrations of lipofectin and 1 μM of the antisense G3139 or the scrambled ISIS 4559 oligonucleotides. Cells were washed with complete medium and then, after 19 h, Western blot (**A**) and Northern blot (**B**) analyses were performed. Anti-Bcl-2 and anti-PKC-α, -β1, -ξ and -ε antibodies were used to measure the protein level. mRNA levels were determined using the PKC-α and GAPDH probes.

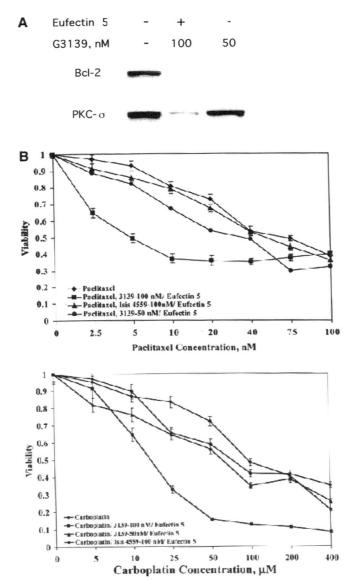

Fig. 9. The carrier Eufectin 5 permits separation of the downregulation of Bcl-2 and PKC-α as a function of oligonucleotide concentration. Twenty-five 10⁴ T24 cells per well were seeded in six-well plates to be 70 to 80% confluent on the next day. Cells were treated for 24 h with preformed complexes of Eufectin 5 (4.75 and 9.5 µg/mL, respectively) and oligonucleotides (50 and 100 nM). Cells were then washed and incubated for 48 h in complete medium. (**A**) The Bcl-2 and PKC-α protein levels were measured by Western blotting, using the respective antibodies. (**B**) The sensitivity of the T24 cells, treated with complexes of Eufectin5/G3139, to Paclitaxel and Carboplatin were also determined by MTT assay.

down-regulated. However, chemosensitivity to both paclitaxel and carboplatin was only observed at the higher concentration. Therefore, a similar situation pertains here as in the case of PKC-α: The down-regulation of the expression of bcl-2 may be necessary, but it is not sufficient to generate a chemosensitive phenotype. Additionally, although it is possible that down-regulation of both PKC-α plus bcl-2 expression are both necessary and sufficient for the generation of chemosensitivity, it is also possible that both are merely markers for other, as yet unknown, events.

Therefore, it appears quite clear that the mechanisms whereby asONs produce sensitivity to chemotherapeutic agents are quite complex, even in tissue culture. However, when used clinically, the pleotropic effects of these molecules may be highly advantageous. Recent completion of a phase II trial in nonsmall-cell lung cancer patients treated with Isis 3521 plus a combination of carboplatin and taxol produced an impressive approx 50% increase in survival (65). Whether this will be duplicated in the ongoing phase III trial is yet to be determined, but it is a priori difficult to understand why down-regulation of a single PKC isoform should have such a profound affect in such a virulent, poorly treatable tumor. Rather, we propose that it is the pleotropic nature of phosphorothioate ONs, acting by mechanisms that have yet to be fully understood in addition to their antisense activity and in combination with cytotoxic chemotherapy, that are creating a desirable clinical endpoint.

REFERENCES

1. Guga P, Koziolkiewicz M, Okruszek A, Stec W. Oligo(nucleoside phosphorothioate)s. In: Stein CA, Krieg A, eds., Applied Antisense Oligonucleotide Technology. New York: Wiley-Liss 1998:23–50.
2. Stec W, Zon G, Egan W, Stec B. Automated solid-phase synthesis, separation, and stereochemistry of phosphorothioate analogues of oligodeoxyribonucleotides. J Am Chem Soc 1984; 106:6077–6080.
3. Jansen B, Wacheck V, Heere-Ress E, et al. Chemosensitisation of malignant melanoma by BCL2 antisense therapy. Lancet 2000; 356:1728–1733.
4. Yuen AR, Halsey J, Fisher GA, et al. Phase I study of an antisense oligonucleotide to protein kinase C-alpha (ISIS 3521/CGP 64128A) in patients with cancer. Clin Cancer Res 1999; 5:3357–3363.
5. Jansen B, Schlagbauer-Wadl H, Brown BD, et al. bcl-2 antisense therapy chemosensitizes human melanoma in SCID mice. Nat Med 1998; 4:232–234.
6. Lebedeva I, Stein CA. Antisense oligonucleotides: promise and reality. Annu Rev Pharmacol Toxicol 2001; 41:403–419.
7. Stein CA. The experimental use of antisense oligonucleotides: a guide for the perplexed. J Clin Invest 2001; 108:641–644.
8. Koziolkiewicz M, Gendaszewska E, Maszewska M, Stein CA, Stec WJ. The mononucleotide-dependent, nonantisense mechanism of action of phosphodiester and phosphorothioate oligonucleotides depends upon the activity of an ecto-5'-nucleotidase. Blood 2001; 98:995–1002.
9. Eder PS, DeVine RJ, Dagle JM, Walder JA. Substrate specificity and kinetics of degradation of antisense oligonucleotides by a 3' exonuclease in plasma. Antisense Res Dev 1991; 1:141–151.

10. Stein CA, Subasinghe C, Shinozuka K, Cohen JS. Physicochemical properties of phosphoro-thioate oligodeoxynucleotides. Nucleic Acids Res 1988; 16:3209–3221.
11. Zhang H, Cook J, Nickel J, et al. Reduction of liver Fas expression by an antisense oligonucle-otide protects mice from fulminant hepatitis. Nat Biotechnol 2000; 18:862–867.
12. Benimetskaya L, Miller P, Benimetsky S, et al. Inhibition of potentially anti-apoptotic pro-teins by antisense protein kinase C-alpha (Isis 3521) and antisense bcl-2 (G3139) phosphoro-thioate oligodeoxynucleotides: relationship to the decreased viability of T24 bladder and PC3 prostate cancer cells. Mol Pharmacol 2001; 60:1296–1307.
13. Lesser DR, Grajkowski A, Kurpiewski MR, Koziolkiewicz M, Stec WJ, Jen-Jacobson L. Stereoselective interaction with chiral phosphorothioates at the central DNA kink of the EcoRI endonuclease-GAATTC complex. J Biol Chem 1992; 267:24810–24818.
14. Marcus-Sekura CJ, Woerner AM, Shinozuka K, Zon G, Quinnan GV, Jr. Comparative inhi-bition of chloramphenicol acetyltransferase gene expression by antisense oligonucleotide analogues having alkyl phosphotriester, methylphosphonate and phosphorothioate linkages. Nucleic Acids Res 1987; 15:5749–5763.
15. Gilar M, Belenky A, Budman Y, Smisek DL, Cohen AS. Impact of 3'-exonuclease stereoselectivity on the kinetics of phosphorothioate oligonucleotide metabolism. Antisense Nucleic Acid Drug Dev 1998; 8:35–42.
16. Koziolkiewicz M, Wojcik M, Kobylanska A, et al. Stability of stereoregular oligo(nucleoside phosphorothioate)s in human plasma: diastereoselectivity of plasma 3'-exonuclease. Antisense Nucleic Acid Drug Dev 1997; 7:43–48.
17. Stec WJ, Grajkowski A, Koziolkiewicz M, Uznanski B. Novel route to oligo(deoxyribo-nucleoside phosphorothioates). Stereocontrolled synthesis of P-chiral oligo(deoxyribo-nucleoside phosphorothioates). Nucleic Acids Res 1991; 19:5883–5888.
18. Wilk A, Grajkowski A, Bull TE, Dixon AM, Freedberg DI, Beaucage SL. Direct assignment of the absolute configuration of a distinct class of deoxyribonucleoside cyclic N-acylphospho-ramidites at phosphorus by M- GOESY nuclear magnetic resonance spectroscopy. J Am Chem Soc 2002; 124:1180–1181.
19. Stec W, Karwowski B, Boczkowska M, et al. Deoxyribonucleoside 3'-O-(2-thio-and 3'-O-(2-oxo"spiro"-4,4-pentamethylene-1,3,2-oxathiaphospholane)s: monomers for stereocontrolled synthesis of oligo(deoxyribonucleoside phosphorothioate)s and chimeric PS/PO oligonucle-otides. J Am Chem Soc 1998; 120:7156–7167.
20. Fennewald SM, Rando RF. Inhibition of high affinity basic fibroblast growth factor binding by oligonucleotides. J Biol Chem 1995; 270:21718–21721.
21. Guvakova MA, Yakubov LA, Vlodavsky I, Tonkinson JL, Stein CA. Phosphorothioate oligodeoxynucleotides bind to basic fibroblast growth factor, inhibit its binding to cell surface receptors, and remove it from low affinity binding sites on extracellular matrix. J Biol Chem 1995; 270:2620–2627.
22. Rockwell P, O'Connor WJ, King K, Goldstein NI, Zhang LM, Stein CA. Cell-surface pertur-bations of the epidermal growth factor and vascular endothelial growth factor receptors by phosphorothioate oligodeoxynucleotides. Proc Natl Acad Sci USA 1997; 94:6523–6528.
23. Khaled Z, Benimetskaya L, Zeltser R, et al. Multiple mechanisms may contribute to the cellular anti-adhesive effects of phosphorothioate oligodeoxynucleotides. Nucleic Acids Res 1996; 24:737–745.
24. Nakajima M, DeChavigny A, Johnson CE, Hamada J, Stein CA, Nicolson GL. Suramin. A potent inhibitor of melanoma heparanase and invasion. J Biol Chem 1991; 266:9661–9666.
25. Miao HQ, Elkin M, Aingorn E, Ishai-Michaeli R, Stein CA, Vlodavsky I. Inhibition of heparanase activity and tumor metastasis by laminarin sulfate and synthetic phosphorothioate oligodeoxynucleotides. Int J Cancer 1999; 83:424–431.
26. Khaled Z, Rideout D, O'Driscoll KR, et al. Effects of suramin-related and other clinically therapeutic polyanions on protein kinase C activity. Clin Cancer Res 1995; 1:113–122.

27. Benimetskaya L, Tonkinson JL, Koziolkiewicz M, et al. Binding of phosphorothioate oligodeoxynucleotides to basic fibroblast growth factor, recombinant soluble CD4, laminin and fibronectin is P- chirality independent. Nucleic Acids Res 1995; 23:4239–4245.

28. Gao WY, Han FS, Storm C, Egan W, Cheng YC. Phosphorothioate oligonucleotides are inhibitors of human DNA polymerases and RNase H: implications for antisense technology. Mol Pharmacol 1992; 41:223–229.

29. Perez JR, Li Y, Stein CA, Majumder S, van Oorschot A, Narayanan R. Sequence-independent induction of Sp1 transcription factor activity by phosphorothioate oligodeoxynucleotides. Proc Natl Acad Sci U S A 1994; 91:5957–5961.

30. Stein CA, Krieg AM. Problems in interpretation of data derived from in vitro and in vivo use of antisense oligodeoxynucleotides. Antisense Res Dev 1994; 4:67–69.

31. Stein CA, Neckers LM, Nair BC, Mumbauer S, Hoke G, Pal R. Phosphorothioate oligo-deoxycytidine interferes with binding of HIV-1 gp120 to CD4. J Acquir Immune Defic Syndr 1991; 4:686–693.

32. Gao WY, Stein CA, Cohen JS, Dutschman GE, Cheng YC. Effect of phosphorothioate homo-oligodeoxynucleotides on herpes simplex virus type 2-induced DNA polymerase. J Biol Chem 1989; 264:11521–11526.

33. Stein CA. Is irrelevant cleavage the price of antisense efficacy? Pharmacol Ther 2000; 85:231–236.

34. Giles RV, Tidd DM. Increased specificity for antisense oligodeoxynucleotide targeting of RNA cleavage by RNase H using chimeric methylphosphonodiester/phosphodiester struc-tures. Nucleic Acids Res 1992a; 20:763–770.

35. Giles RV, Tidd DM. Enhanced RNase H activity with methylphosphonodiester/phosphodiester chimeric antisense oligodeoxynucleotides. Anticancer Drug Des 1992b; 7:37–48.

36. Walder RY, Walder JA. Role of RNase H in hybrid-arrested translation by antisense oligo-nucleotides. Proc Natl Acad Sci USA 1988; 85:5011–5015.

37. Minshull J, Hunt T. The use of single-stranded DNA and RNase H to promote quantitative 'hybrid arrest of translation' of mRNA/DNA hybrids in reticulocyte lysate cell-free transla-tions. Nucleic Acids Res 1986; 14:6433–6451.

38. Cazenave C, Loreau N, Thuong NT, Toulme JJ, Helene C. Enzymatic amplification of trans-lation inhibition of rabbit beta-globin mRNA mediated by anti-messenger oligodeoxynucleo-tides covalently linked to intercalating agents. Nucleic Acids Res 1987; 15:4717–4736.

39. Monia BP, Lesnik EA, Gonzalez C, et al. Evaluation of 2'-modified oligonucleotides containing 2'-deoxy gaps as antisense inhibitors of gene expression. J Biol Chem 1993; 268:14514–14522.

40. Mir KU, Southern EM. Determining the influence of structure on hybridization using oligo-nucleotide arrays. Nat Biotechnol 1999; 17:788–792.

41. Dean NM, McKay R. Inhibition of protein kinase C-alpha expression in mice after systemic administration of phosphorothioate antisense oligodeoxynucleotides. Proc Natl Acad Sci USA 1994; 91:11762–11766.

42. Dean NM, McKay R, Condon TP, Bennett CF. Inhibition of protein kinase C-alpha expression in human A549 cells by antisense oligonucleotides inhibits induction of intercellular adhesion molecule 1 (ICAM-1) mRNA by phorbol esters. J Biol Chem 1994; 269:16416–16424.

43. Benimetskaya L, Takle GB, Vilenchik M, Lebedeva I, Miller P, Stein CA. Cationic porphy-rins: novel delivery vehicles for antisense oligodeoxynucleotides. Nucleic Acids Res 1998; 26:5310–5317.

44. Gee JE, Robbins I, van der Laan AC, et al. Assessment of high-affinity hybridization, RNase H cleavage, and covalent linkage in translation arrest by antisense oligonucleotides. Antisense Nucleic Acid Drug Dev 1998; 8:103–111.

45. Heidenreich O, Gryaznov S, Nerenberg M. RNase H-independent antisense activity of oligo-
    nucleotide N3 '—> P5 ' phosphoramidates. Nucleic Acids Res 1997; 25:776–780.
46. Furdon PJ, Dominski Z, Kole R. RNase H cleavage of RNA hybridized to oligonucleotides
    containing methylphosphonate, phosphorothioate and phosphodiester bonds. Nucleic Acids
    Res 1989; 17:9193–9204.
47. Giles RV, Spiller DG, Grzybowski J, Clark RE, Nicklin P, Tidd DM. Selecting optimal
    oligonucleotide composition for maximal antisense effect following streptolysin O-mediated
    delivery into human leukaemia cells. Nucleic Acids Res 1998; 26:1567–1575.
48. Bonham MA, Brown S, Boyd AL, et al. An assessment of the antisense properties of RNase
    H-competent and steric-blocking oligomers. Nucleic Acids Res 1995; 23:1197–1203.
49. Chiang MY. Chan H, Zounes MA, Freier SM, Lima WF, Bennett CF. Antisense oligonucle-
    otides inhibit intercellular adhesion molecule 1 expression by two distinct mechanisms. J Biol
    Chem 1991; 266:18162–18171.
50. Liebhaber SA, Cash FE, Shakin SH. Translationally associated helix-destabilizing activity in
    rabbit reticulocyte lysate. J Biol Chem 1984; 259:15597–15602.
51. Dias N, Dheur S, Nielsen PE, et al. Antisense PNA tridecamers targeted to the coding region
    of Ha-ras mRNA arrest polypeptide chain elongation. J Mol Biol 1999; 294:403–416.
52. Baker BF, Lot SS, Condon TP, et al. 2'-O-(2-Methoxy)ethyl-modified anti-intercellular adhe-
    sion molecule 1 (ICAM-1) oligonucleotides selectively increase the ICAM-1 mRNA level and
    inhibit formation of the ICAM-1 translation initiation complex in human umbilical vein en-
    dothelial cells. J Biol Chem 1997; 272:11994–2000.
53. Gray GD, Basu S, Wickstrom E. Transformed and immortalized cellular uptake of
    oligodeoxynucleoside phosphorothioates, 3'-alkylamino oligodeoxynucleotides, 2'-O-methyl
    oligoribonucleotides, oligodeoxynucleoside methylphosphonates, and peptide nucleic acids.
    Biochem Pharmacol 1997; 53:1465–1476.
54. Braasch DA, Corey DR. Locked nucleic acid (LNA): fine-tuning the recognition of DNA and
    RNA. Chem Biol 2001; 8:1–7.
55. Koshkin AA, Singh SK, Nielsen PE, et al. LNA (locked nucleic acids): synthesis of the
    adenine, cytosine, guanine, 5-methylcytosine. thymine and uracil bicyclonucleoside mono-
    mers, oligomerisation and unprecedented nucleic acid recognition. Tetrahedron 1998;
    54:3607–3630.
56. Shen LX, Kandimalla ER, Agrawal S. Impact of mixed-backbone oligonucleotides on target
    binding affinity and target cleaving specificity and selectivity by Escherichia coli RNase H.
    Bioorg Med Chem 1998; 6:1695–1705.
57. Agrawal S, Jiang Z, Zhao Q, et al. Mixed-backbone oligonucleotides as second generation
    antisense oligonucleotides: in vitro and in vivo studies. Proc Natl Acad Sci USA 1997;
    94:2620–2625.
58. Giles RV, Ruddell CJ, Spiller DG, Green JA, Tidd DM. Single base discrimination for ribo-
    nuclease H-dependent antisense effects within intact human leukaemia cells. Nucleic Acids
    Res 1995; 23:954–961.
59. Larrouy B, Boiziau C, Sproat B, Toulme JJ. RNase H is responsible for the non-specific
    inhibition of in vitro translation by 2'-O-alkyl chimeric oligonucleotides: high affinity or
    selectivity, a dilemma to design antisense oligomers. Nucleic Acids Res 1995; 23:3434–3440.
60. Ma M, Benimetskaya L, Lebedeva I, Dignam J, Takle G, Stein CA. Intracellular mRNA
    cleavage induced through activation of RNase P by nuclease-resistant external guide
    sequences. Nat Biotechnol 2000; 18:58–61.
61. Ma MY, Jacob-Samuel B, Dignam JC, Pace U, Goldberg AR, George ST. Nuclease-resistant
    external guide sequence-induced cleavage of target RNA by human ribonuclease P. Antisense
    Nucleic Acid Drug Dev 1998; 8:415–426.
62. Altman S. RNA enzyme-directed gene therapy. Proc Natl Acad Sci USA 1993; 90:10898–10900.
63. Forster AC, Altman S. External guide sequences for an RNA enzyme. Science 1990;
    249:783–786.

64. Yuan Y, Hwang ES, Altman S. Targeted cleavage of mRNA by human RNase P. Proc Natl Acad Sci USA 1992; 89:8006–8010.
65. Evans TL, Lynch TJ, Jr. Lung cancer. Oncologist 2001; 6:407–414.

15 Antisense Protein Kinase A-RIα Restores Normal Signal Transduction Signatures to Inhibit Tumor Growth

Yoon S. Cho-Chung, MD, PhD

CONTENTS

1. INTRODUCTION

During the early steps required to activate adenosine 3',5'-cyclic monophosphate (cAMP) signaling, cAMP binds its receptor, cAMP-dependent protein kinase (PKA) *(1)*, and induces reversible phosphorylation of protein substrates that regulate a vast number of cellular processes, including cell growth and differentiation. Researchers interested in the regulation of cell growth by cAMP have focused on the two isoforms of PKA, type I (PKA-I) and type II (PKA-II), which differ in their regulatory subunits, RI and RII, respectively. Recent experimental evidence has shown that the balanced, intracellular expression between the two isoforms may play a critical role in the control of cell growth and differentiation, pointing to distinct functions for PKA-I and PKA-II. PKA-I is only transiently overexpressed in normal cells in response to the physiological stimu-

From: *Cancer Drug Discovery and Development:*
Nucleic Acid Therapeutics in Cancer
Edited by: A. M. Gewirtz © Humana Press Inc., Totowa, NJ

lation of cell proliferation *(2,3)*. However, this isoform is constitutively overexpressed in cancer cells and associated with a poor prognosis in human cancers of different cell types *(4–8)*. Conversely, PKA-II is preferentially expressed in normal, differentiated tissues *(8–10)*.

This review describes the influence of each regulatory subunit on the circuitry of cAMP signaling in cell growth and differentiation. Experimental approaches described here include antisense oligonucleotides, gene transfer, and gene-expression profiling. These approaches not only provide the molecular tools to critically assess the role of cAMP signaling in cancer genesis and progression, but they also contribute to the discovery of novel, target-based drugs for the treatment of cancer.

2. RIα OVEREXPRESSION AND MITOGENIC SIGNAL

Increased expression of RI has been associated with both chemical and viral carcinogenesis and with oncogene-induced cell transformation. The initiation stage of dimethylbenz (a) anthracene-induced mammary carcinogenesis in rats *(11)*, the incidence of gastric adenocarcinoma in rats by *N*-methyl-*N*(-nitrosguanine, and the trophic action of gastrin on gastric carcinoma production *(12)* correlate with a sharp increase in RI and PKA-I expression. Spontaneously transformed 3T3 cells and cells transformed with SV40 or with methylcholanthrene express both PKA-I and PKA-II, with an increased level of RI *(13,14)*, although PKA-I is not normally expressed in normal 3T3 cells. However, the level of total PKA activity in transformed cells is equivalent to that of normal cells. A similar increase in RI and PKA-I expression has been shown in rat 3Y1 cells transformed by human adenovirus type 12 *(15)* A marked increase in RI expression, with a concomitant decrease in RII expression, has also been detected in Ha-MuSV-transformed NIH/3T3 clone 13-3B-4 cells *(16)*, in rat (NRK) kidney cells transformed with transforming growth factor (TGF) or *v-Ki-ras* oncogene *(17)*, in TGF-induced transformation of mouse mammary epithelial cells *(18)*, and in MCF-10A HE *(19)*, a human mammary cell line transformed by point mutations in the *c-Ha-ras* and *c-erbB-2* proto-oncogenes. Importantly, expression of the RIα subunit of PKA is increased in various primary human tumors and cell lines, including cancers of the breast *(4,5,20)*, ovary *(6,7)*, lung *(21)*, and colon *(22–24)*.

Overexpression of the RIα subunit also has been correlated with multidrug resistance (MDR) *(25)*, the regulation of cytochrome C through its interaction with CoxVb *(26)*, and the ligand-activated epidermal growth factor receptor (EGFR) complex through its interaction with the Grb2 adaptor protein *(27)*. Thus, overexpression of RIα may deregulate a multitude of cellular functions that regulate cell growth and MDR. These results all suggest that RI may mediate various mitogenic stimuli and thus represent a potential target for the pharmacological control of cell proliferation.

3. ANTISENSE INHIBITION OF RIα

3.1. Blockade of Tumor Growth

Nucleic acid therapeutics represent a direct genetic approach to cancer treatment. Such an approach takes advantage of mechanisms that activate genes known to confer a growth advantage to neoplastic cells *(28)*. The ability to block the expression of these genes allows the exploration of normal growth regulation.

Overexpression of RIα in cancer cells that have "inborn" growth-advantageous properties, such as hormone-, serum-, and anchorage-independent growth, has no apparent effect on the rate of cell proliferation *(29)*. However, in nontransformed cells such as FRTL5 rat thyroid cells and immortalized human mammary epithelial cells (MCF-10A), RIα overexpression mimics the effect of hormone and serum supplements on cell growth and cell-cycle progression in tissue culture *(2,3)*.

One of the critical structural differences between RI and RII is the presence of an autophosphorylation site in RII at the R·C junction*(30)*. An autophosphorylation site has been introduced into human RIα at alanine 99 via a single nucleotide change, G→T, that replaces this alanine with serine. Overexpression of this mutant, RIα-P, in MCF-7 breast cancer cells inhibits growth and induces apoptosis *(31)*. Cells overexpressing RIα-P also require a higher concentration of cAMP to activate endogenous PKA than do cells overexpressing wild-type RIα. Additionally, RIα-P downregulates PKA-II) *31)*, unlike wild-type RIα, which cannot downregulate PKA-II by overexpression *(29,32)*. The dominant activity of RIα-P may arise from the ability of this mutant to trap endogenous, wild-type RIα into inactive dimers, blocking PKA-I activity and thereby inhibiting growth.

The possibility that RI is a positive regulator of cancer cell growth has been further explored using the antisense strategy. A synthetic, RIα antisense, unmodified oligodeoxynucleotide (ODN) corresponding to the N-terminal seven codons of human RIα (15–30 μM) downregulates RIα and upregulates the competitor molecule RIIβ, and it inhibits growth in breast (MCF-7), colon (LS-174T), gastric carcinoma (TMK-1), neuroblastoma (SK-N-SH) cells *(33)*, and HL-60 leukemia cells *(34)* with no sign of cytotoxicity. Furthermore, treatment with an RIα antisense phosphorothioate oligodeoxynucleotide (PS-ODN) at a much lower concentration (6 μM) brings about a marked reduction in RIα levels with a concomitant increase in RIIβ levels *(33)*. Strikingly, a single injection of RIα antisense PS-ODN targeted against codons 8–13 of human RIα results in the reduction of RIα expression and in sustained growth inhibition of LS-174T colon carcinoma in nude mice at up to 14 d of examination *(35)*. Tumor cells behave like untransformed cells by making less PKA-I *(35)*.

3.2. Second Generation RNA-DNA Antisense ODN Is the Better CHOICE: Target-Specific, Nonimmune Stimulatory and Minimum Side Effects

To address the issue of nonspecific toxicity and side effects associated with antisense PS-ODNs, the polyanionic nature *(36)* of the antisense RIα PS-ODN has been minimized, and the immunostimulatory GCGT motif *(37)* has been blocked in a second-generation RNA–DNA RIα antisense *(38)*. These RNA–DNA ODNs have improved antisense activity over the PS-ODNs *(39,40)*, are more resistant to nucleases, form more stable duplexes with RNA than the parental PS-ODN *(39,41)*, and retain the capability to induce RNase H *(39)*. Thus, in addition to reducing nonspecific effects, the RNA–DNA RIα antisense ODN facilitates the exploration of sequence-specific antisense effects *(38)*. This modulation ultimately inhibits growth and induces apoptosis in various cancer cell lines and in tumors in nude mice *(9,38,42–49)*.

The target specificity of RIα antisense has been thoroughly addressed. Pulse-chase experiments have revealed that RIα has a relatively short half-life: 17 h in control cells and 13 h in antisense-treated cells (i.e., LS-174T colon carcinoma cells) *(45)*. The short half-life of RIα, along with its message down-regulation, is consistent with the rapid RIα down-regulation observed in antisense-treated tumors *(35)*. Additionally, levels of RIIβ protein increase because of a longer half-life (about a 5.5-fold increase over that in untreated control cells) *(45)*, leading to a decrease in the PKA-I to PKA-II ratio in tumor cells *(35)*. The half-lives of RIIα and Cα remain unchanged in antisense-treated cells *(45)*. RIα antisense-induced stabilization of the RIIβ protein is consistent with results in RIβ and RIIβ knockout mice, in which a compensatory, stabilization-induced elevation of RIα appears in tissues that normally express the β isoforms of the R subunit *(50)*. These results show a clear, target-specific correlation between growth inhibition induced by RIα antisense and RIα down-regulation.

3.3. Inhibition of Signaling Cascade Is Cell Specific

The effects of the RIα antisense RNA–DNA ODN on the cAMP-signaling cascade depend on the expression of PKA-I and PKA-II in the cell. In LS-174T colon cancer cells and in LNCaP prostate cancer cells, in which both PKA-I and PKA-II are expressed *(29)*, the antisense-directed loss of RIα results in the expected compensatory stabilization of the RIIβ protein, again because RIIβ's half-life is lengthened *(45)*. Treatment with the antisense ODN also triggers an increase in the activity of PDE4 *(38)*, a cAMP-inducible enzyme *(51,52)*, and the nuclear translocation of the PKA Cα subunit *(53)* in the absence of increased cellular cAMP. Thus, the loss of RIα activates cAMP signaling by activating PKA-I and bypassing adenylate cyclase. However, in the case of HCT-15 MDR colon carcinoma cells, in which PKA-I is primarily expressed *(54)*, the antisense-directed loss of RIα shortens the half-life of Cα *(38)*. This leads to a reduction in cAMP signaling as evidenced by reduced PDE4 activity *(38)*. These results are consistent with those observed in S49 lymphoma cells, which only express PKA-I *(55)*. The RI subunit becomes much more labile in mutant cells lacking a functional C subunit than in wild-type cells, and in cells treated with cAMP analogs than in untreated control cells *(55)*.

These results can be interpreted in the context of cAMP response element-directed transcription. PKA activates the transactivation activity of cAMP response element-binding protein (CREB) *(56)* by phosphorylating Ser 133 *(57)*. Phosphorylation at this amino acid is also crucial for growth-factor induction of *c-fos* transcription *(58)*. In transformed cells, growth-factor-mediated phospho-rylation of CREB may supersede that mediated by PKA and therefore stimulate cell growth. However, upon RIα antisense treatment, activated PKA, which is the released Cα subunit, may augment Cα-mediated CREB-phosphorylation, causing a switch in the mechanism of CREB phosphorylation from one mediated by growth factors to one mediated by PKA. This switch might inhibit growth-factor signals and, ultimately, cell growth in LS-174T and LNCaP cancer cells *(38)*. In HCT-15 MDR cells, the RIα antisense, RNA–DNA ODN-directed destabilization of Cα may simply turn off transactivation of CRE, AP-1, and Sp-1, which are commonly upregulated in HCT-15 MDR cells *(59)*, and thereby inhibit cell growth *(38)*. The oral efficacy *(49)* and the growth inhibition exerted by RIα antisense RNA–DNA second-generation ODN in cancer cells of a variety of cell types *(9,38,42–49)* support efforts to test the effects of this antisense ODN on tumors in a clinical setting (GEM 231, an RIα antisense RNA–DNA second-generation ODN) *(60)*.

4. RIIβ OVEREXPRESSION AND ISOZYME DISTRIBUTION

4.1. RIIβ Overexpression Induces Reverted Phenotype

The RIIβ subunit is essential for cAMP-induced growth inhibition and differ-entiation in cancer cells. An RIIβ antisense ODN blocks the growth inhibition and differentiation induced by cAMP. Cells become refractory to the cAMP stimulus and continue to grow in the presence or absence of a cAMP analog *(61)*.

The relationship between RIIβ expression and malignancy has been tested using vector-mediated overexpression of RIIβ. Overexpression of RIIβ inhibits growth, with no sign of toxicity, in a variety of cancer cell types, including SK-N-SH neuroblastoma, MCF-7 breast carcinoma, *Ki-ras*-transformed NIH/3T3 clone DT *(62,63)*, HL-60 leukemia cells *(63)*, and PC12 mutant A-126 cells *(64)*. SK-N-SH, DT, and A-126 cells also display striking changes in morphology. Cells become flat and exhibit an increased ratio of cytoplasm to nucleus *(62–64)*. Cells exposed to RIα antisense ODN exhibit similar morphology *(34)*. In SK-N-

SH and HL-60 cells, overexpression of RIIβ directly induces growth arrest and reversion of the transformed phenotype; no further treatment with cAMP analogs is required. These results suggest that the RIIβ subunit may act as a tumor suppressor protein that inhibits growth and promotes differentiation and reverse transformation.

RIIβ activates transcription by binding to the CRE *(65)*. cAMP enhances the ability of RIIβ to bind the CRE, and the mutant RIIβ-P, in which the auto-phosphorylation site (Ser 114) has been changed to alanine, is incapable of binding the CRE and inefficient in activating transcription *(65)*. Cells over-expressing RIIβ-P behave as transformed cells *(29,66)* and exhibit an increase in a novel, 53-kDa RIIβ protein species that is not detected in parental cells *(29)*. Decreased RIα levels are also detected in these cells.

4.2. Preferential Formation of PKA-II Over PKA-I Formation in Intact Cells

Overexpression of the RII subunit induces a striking shift in PKA isozyme distribution by reducing PKA-I levels and increasing PKA-II levels in LS-174T colon carcinoma cells *(29)*. PKA-I levels are almost completely eliminated in cells overexpressing RIIβ and RIIβ-P, and different species of PKA-II, which do not appear in parental cells or in cells overexpressing RIIα, are detected in these cells. In contrast, PKA-II levels are unaltered in cells overexpressing RIα and in cells overexpressing Cα. These data suggest that the R and C subunits are in equilibrium between PKA-I and PKA-II and that PKA-II formation is highly favored in intact cells.

This preferential formation of PKA-II is not limited to LS-174T cells; such a preference has also been demonstrated in *ras*-transformed NIH3T3 cells and in AtT20 pituitary cells *(32)*. Most likely, RIIα and Cα associate preferentially in LS-174T cells, and PKA-I is formed only if the C subunit is present in excess over RIIα. Excess, free RIα may be degraded; therefore, an increase in RIα or PKA-I cannot occur in cells overexpressing RIα even though RIα mRNA increases *(29)*.

4.3. Preferential Formation of PKA-I in Primary Human Tumors

Evidence has shown a correlation between the ratio of PKA-1 to PKA-II and ontogenic development and differentiation *(67,68)*. The ratio in renal cell carcinomas is about twice that in renal cortex, although total soluble PKA activity is similar in both tissues *(69)*. Surgical specimens of Wilms' tumor exhibit a ratio that is twice that found in normal tissue, and the ratio of RI to RII in tumors is more than three times that in normal tissue *(70)*. In a study of rat pituitary tumors, RII appears at lower levels in nuclei isolated from tumors than in normal tissue *(71)*. In the neoplastically transformed BT5C glioma cell line, the ratio of PKA-I to PKA-II is significantly higher than in normal fetal brain cells, but the R and C subunits of protein kinase are expressed to a similar degree in both cell lines *(72)*.

Normal and malignant osteoblasts also differ in their isozyme response to hormones, with a relative predominance of PKA-I activation in malignant cells and of PKA-II in normal cells *(73)*. In addition, increased expression of PKA-I, compared with PKA-II, has also been correlated with the MDR of cancer cells *(25,59)*.

The increased level of stable PKA-I found in primary tumors, in contrast to the favored formation of PKA-II over PKA-I demonstrated by overexpression of the wild-type R subunits, suggests an intrinsic structural alteration in R subunits in tumor cells, possibly at the site of interaction between the R subunit and the C subunit. However, no such mutant of the R subunit has been identified in cancer cells. Nevertheless, the results mentioned above suggest that abnormal expression of R-subunit isoforms of PKA is involved in neoplastic transformation and that suppression of RIα/PKA-I or induction of RIIβ/PKA-IIβ can restore growth control in transformed cells.

5. DEFINING ANTISENSE EFFECTS THROUGH CDNA MICROARRAY ANALYSIS

A cDNA microarray *(74)* has been used to investigate sequence-specific effects of antisense RIα on global gene expression. *(75*; Fig. 1*)* To verify the specificity of the antisense effects on gene-expression signatures, two distinct antisense, PS-ODNs—one with the immunostimulatory CpG motif, and the other without the immunostimulatory motif—and a second-generation RNA–DNA antisense ODN, which targets human or mouse RIα mRNA, are used *(75)*. Additionally, this study shows the expression profile in cells endogenously overexpressing the RIα antisense gene. This system avoids the problems inherent in ODN treatment, namely, the delivery and stability of the ODN.

The results show that in a sequence-specific manner, antisense targeted to PKA RIα alters expression of the clusters of coordinately expressed genes. The DNA microarray technology has made possible, for the first time, the demonstration that the antisense RIα in its sequence-specific manner, is able to modulate a wide set of genes related to cell proliferation and transformation vs others involved in growth arrest and differentiation. Thus, the antisense-directed depletion of the RIα subunit of PKA modulates the signal transduction signatures of multiple pathways beyond that of cAMP pathway. This leads to a reverted tumor phenotype in which the tumor stops growing. This approach has, therefore, confirmed and extended the findings generated by studies of a decade that are based on experiments conducted with the classical methodologies of biochemistry and molecular biology, and translational approaches.

6. PERSPECTIVE

Antisense ODNs can specifically inhibit gene expression, and they can ultimately affect abnormal cell proliferation. The down-regulation of genes that

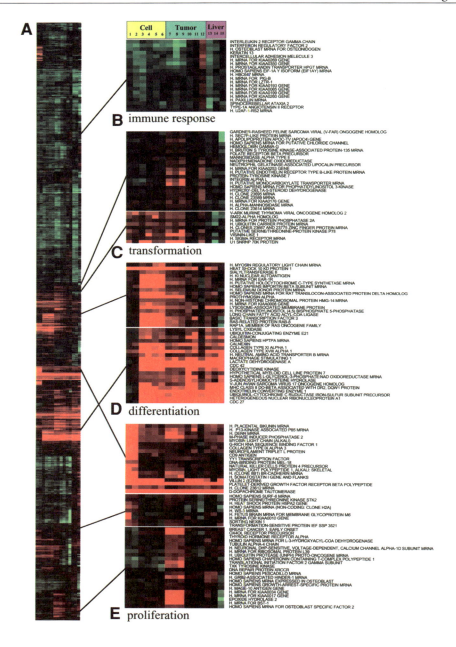

Fig. 1. Molecular portrait of the reverted phenotype (flat) of PC3M cells and tumors treated with antisense RIα. Data from control oligodeoxynucleotide (ODN)-treated cells, antisense ODN/gene-treated cells, untreated control cells, antisense ODN- or control ODN-treated tumors, control tumors, and host livers were combined and clustered. Clus-

contribute to cancer progression has been the goal of antisense research, with the expectation that such an approach may lead to a selective or preferential inhibition of tumor growth without harming normal cell growth.

The positive and negative regulatory functions of cAMP in eukaryotic cell growth appear to be governed by the predominance of either one of the two types of PKA, type I, and type II, present in the cell. Modulation of the R subunit expression using antisense strategy, the type-1 PKA activator 8-Cl-cAMP, or retroviral vector-mediated gene transfer has shown that two isoforms of cAMP receptor proteins, the RIα and RIIβ regulatory subunits, of the type I and type II PKA, respectively, have opposite roles in cancer cell growth. RIα appears to promote cell growth, and RIIβ inhibits growth and induces differentiation.

Gene-expression profiling, using cDNA microarrays, places cAMP and PKA at the heart of the signal-transduction circuitry that controls cell growth and differentiation. In a sequence-specific manner, the antisense depletion of RIα coordinately up-regulated a specific subset of genes (the differentiation signature) and down-regulated another subset (the proliferation signature) in tumor cells. These signatures were quiescent and unaltered in the host livers of antisense-treated animals. Thus, the microarrays painted a molecular portrait of the antisense-induced, reverted phenotype of tumors that stop growing. cDNA microarrays thus provided documentary proof that the RIα regulatory subunit of PKA functions as a positive regulator of tumor growth.

The RIα antisense induces growth inhibition in a variety of cancers of epithelial cell origin as well as in leukemia cells supporting its therapeutic application

---

Fig. 1. *(continued from previous page)* ter analysis was performed on Z-transformed microarray data by using two separate programs available as shareware from Michael Eisen's lab (http://rana.lbl.gov). Each gene is represented by a single row of colored boxes; each experimental sample is represented by a single column: columns 1 and 2, untreated control cells; columns 3 and 4, antisense RNA/DNA hybrid ODN-treated cells; columns 5 and 6, antisense gene overexpressing cells; columns 7 and 8, untreated control tumors; column 9, control ODN-treated tumor; column 10, antisense RNA–DNA ODN-treated tumor; column 11, mouse antisense PS-ODN-treated tumor; column 12, antisense PS-ODN-treated tumor; column 13, antisense PS-ODN-treated liver; column 14, antisense RNA–DNA ODN-treated liver; column 15, untreated control liver. The entire cluster image is shown in **A**. Full gene names are shown for representative clusters containing functionally related genes involved in (**B**) immune response, (**C**) transformation, (**D**) differentiation, and (**E**) proliferation. These clusters also contain uncharacterized genes and named genes not involved in these processes. The size of the tumors compared with untreated (saline injected) control tumors were 42, 63, 56, and 98% after 4 d of treatment with antisense RNA–DNA ODN, PS-ODN, mouse PS-ODN, and control ODN, respectively. There was no sign of systemic toxicity in treated animals, and the size of the liver and spleen remained unchanged *(75)*.

toward a broad spectrum of cancer. Importantly, the RIα antisense is also a potent antitumor agent for MDR tumors. Future clinical applications of RIα antisense oligonucleotide may include its combination with 8-Cl-cAMP, the PKA-I down-regulator; differentiation agents, such as retinoic acid; monoclonal antibodies targeting growth-factor receptors; conventional chemotherapeutic agents; and immune-modulating oligonucleotides such as CpG oligos. Importantly, it has been demonstrated that RIα antisense does not interfere with but shows coopera-tive/synergistic growth-inhibitory effect when combined with cytotoxic drugs.

The diversity and complexity of the cAMP signaling are highly dependent on different stages of normal cellular development and differentiation, and such signaling is disrupted in an abnormal physiology such as cancer. An intervention targeting cAMP signaling may therefore provide a more selective and effective method of restraining tumor cell growth without affecting normal cell growth.

The demonstration of the central role of PKA type-I as a protein-integrating multiple signaling pathway in the cancer cells clearly supports the use of the selective inhibitors of PKA type-I, originally devised as investigative tools, as now potential targeted therapeutic to treat cancer. Both antisense RIα (GEM231, Hybridon, Inc.) and 8-Cl-cAMP (ICN Pharm, Inc.) are currently undergoing clinical phase I and II studies.

ACKNOWLEDGMENT

The author thanks Dr. Frances McFarland of Palladian Partners, Inc., who provided editorial support under contract no. NO2-BC-76212/C2700212 with the National Cancer Institute.

REFERENCES

1. Krebs EG. Protein kinases. Curr Top Cell Regul 1972; 5:99–133.
2. Tortora G, Pepe S, Bianco C, et al. The RIα subunit of protein kinase A controls serum dependency and entry into cell cycle of human mammary epithelial cells. Oncogene 1994; 9:3233–3240.
3. Tortora G, Pepe S, Cirafici AM, et al. Thyroid-stimulating hormone-regulated growth and cell cycle distribution of thyroid cells involve type I isozyme of cyclic AMP- dependent protein kinase. Cell Growth Differ 1993; 4:359–365.
4. Miller WR, Hulme MJ, Cho-Chung YS, Elton RA. Types of cyclic AMP binding proteins in human breast cancers. Eur J Cancer 1993; 29A:989–991.
5. Miller WR, Watson DMA, Jack W, Chetty U, Elton RA. Tumor cyclic AMP binding proteins: An independent prognostic factor for disease recurrence and survival in breast cancer. Breast Cancer Res Treat 1993; 26:89–94.
6. Simpson BJB, Ramage AD, Hulme MJ, et al. Cyclic adenosine 3',5'-monophosphate-binding proteins in human ovarian cancer: Correlations with clinicapachological features. Clin Cancer Res 1996; 2:201–206.
7. McDaid HM, Cairns MT, Atkinson RI, et al. Increased expression of the RIα subunit of the cAMP-dependent protein kinase A is associated with advanced stage of ovarian cancer. Br J Cancer 1999; 79:933–939.

8. Cho-Chung YS, Pepe S, Clair T, Budillon A, Nesterova M. cAMP-dependent protein kinase: role in normal and malignant growth. Crit Rev Oncol Hematol 1995; 21:33–61.
9. Cho-Chung YS, Nesterova M, Pepe S, et al. Antisense DNA-targeting protein kinase A-RIA subunit: a novel approach to cancer treatment. Front Biosci 1999; 4:D898–907.
10. Tortora G, Ciardiello F. Targeting of epidermal growth factor receptor and protein kinase A: molecular basis and therapeutic applications. Ann Oncol 2000; 11:777–783.
11. Cho-Chung YS, Clair T, Shepheard C. Anticarcinogenic effect of N6,O2-dibutyryl cyclic adenosine 3':5'-monophosphate on 7,12-dimethylbenz(α)anthracene mammary tumor induction in the rat and its relationship to cyclic adenosine 3':5'-monophosphate metabolism and protein kinase. Cancer Res 1983; 43:2736–2740.
12. Yasui W, Tahara E. Effect of gastrin on gastric mucosal cyclic adenosine 3',5'-monophosphate-dependent protein kinase activity in rat stomach carcinogenesis induced by N-methyl-N-nitro-N-nitrosoguanidine. Cancer Res 1985; 45:4763–4767.
13. Gharrett AJ, Malkinson AM, Sheppard JR. Cyclic AMP-dependent protein kinases from normal and SV40-transformed 3T3 cells. Nature 1976; 264:673–675.
14. Wehner JM, Malkinson AM, Wiser MF, Sheppard JR. Cyclic AMP-dependent protein kinases from Balb 3T3 cells and other 3T3 derived lines. J Cell Physiol 1981; 108:175–184.
15. Ledinko N, Chan I-JAD. Increase in type I cyclic adenosine 3',5'-monophosphate-dependent protein kinase activity and specific accumulation of type I regulatory subunits in adenovirus type 12-transformed cells. Cancer Res 1984; 44:2622–2627.
16. Clair T, Ally S, Tagliaferri P, Robins RK, Cho-Chung YS. Site-selective cAMP analogs induce nuclear translocation of the RII cAMP receptor protein in Ha-MuSV-transformed NIH/3T3 cells. FEBS Lett 1987; 224:377–384.
17. Tortora G, Ciardiello F, Ally S, Clair T, Salomon DS, Cho-Chung YS. Site-selective 8-chloroadenosine 3',5'-cyclic monophosphate inhibits transformation and transforming growth factor alpha production in Ki- ras-transformed rat fibroblasts. FEBS Lett 1989; 242:363–367.
18. Ciardiello F, Tortora G, Kim N, et al. 8-Chloro-cAMP inhibits transforming growth factor a transformation of mammary epithelial cells by restoration of the normal mRNA patterns for cAMP-dependent protein kinase regulatory subunit isoforms which show disruption upon transformation. J Biol Chem 1990; 265:1016–1020.
19. Ciardiello F, Pepe S, Bianco C, et al. Down-regulation of RIα subunit of cAMP-dependent protein kinase induces growth inhibition of human mammary epithelial cells transformed by c-Ha-ras and c-erbB-2 proto-oncogenes. Int J Cancer 1993; 53:438–443.
20. Handschin JS, Eppenberger U. Altered cellular ratio of type I and type II cyclic AMP-dependent protein kinase in human mammary tumors. FEBS Lett 1979; 106:301–304.
21. Young MRI, Montpettit M, Lozano Y, et al. Regulation of Lewis lung carcinoma invasion and metastasis by protein kinase A. Int J Cancer 1995; 61:104–109.
22. Bradbury AW, Carter DC, Miller WR, Cho-Chung YS, Clair T. Protein kinase A (PK-A) regulatory subunit expression in colorectal cancer and related mucosa. Br J Cancer 1994; 69:738–742.
23. Bold RJ, Alpard S, Ishizuka J, Townsend CM, Jr., Thompson JC. Growth-regulatory effect of gastrin on human colon cancer cell lines is determined by protein kinase a isoform content. Regul Pept 1994; 53:61–70.
24. Gordge PC, Hulme MJ, Clegg RA, Miller WR. Elevation of protein kinase A and protein kinase C activities in malignant as compared with normal human breast tissue. Eur J Cancer 1996; 32A:2120–2126.
25. Yokozaki H, Budillon A, Clair GT, et al. 8-chloroadenosine 3',5'-monophosphate as a novel modulator of multidrug resistance. Int J Oncol 1993; 3:423–430.
26. Yang WL, Iacono L, Tang WM, Chin KV. Novel function of the regulatory subunit of protein kinase A: regulation of cytochrome c oxidase activity and cytochrome c release. Biochemistry 1998; 37:14175–14180.

27. Tortora G, Damiano V, Bianco C, et al. The RIa subunit of protein kinase A (PKA) binds to Grb2 and allows PKA interaction with the activated EGF-receptor. Oncogene 1997; 14:923–928.
28. Zamecnik P, Stephenson M. Inhibition of Rous sarcoma virus replication and cell transformation by a specific oligodeoxynucleotide. Proc Natl Acad Sci USA 1978; 75:280–284.
29. Nesterova MV, Yokozaki H, McDuffie L, Cho-Chung YS. Overexpression of RIIβ regulatory subunit of protein kinase A in human colon carcinoma cell induces growth arrest and phenotypic changes that are abolished by site-directed mutation of RIIβ. Eur J Cancer 1996; 253:486–494.
30. Taylor SS, Bubis J, Toner-Webb J, et al. cAMP-dependent protein kinase: prototype for a family of enzymes. FASEB J 1988; 2:2677–2685.
31. Lee GR, Kim SN, Noguchi K, Park SD, Hong SH, Cho-Chung YS. Ala99ser mutation in RI alpha regulatory subunit of protein kinase A causes reduced kinase activation by cAMP and arrest of hormone- dependent breast cancer cell growth. Mol Cell Biochem 1999; 195:77–86.
32. McKnight GS, Clegg CH, Uhler MD, et al. Analysis of the cAMP-dependent protein kinase system using molecular genetic approaches. Recent Prog Horm Res 1988; 44:307–335.
33. Yokozaki H, Budillon A, Tortora G, et al. An antisense oligodeoxynucleotide that depletes RIα subunit of cyclic AMP-dependent protein kinase induces growth inhibition in human cancer cells. Cancer Res 1993; 53:868–872.
34. Tortora G, Yokozaki H, Pepe S, Clair T, Cho-Chung YS. Differentiation of HL-60 leukemia cells by type I regulatory subunit antisense oligodeoxynucleotide of cAMP-dependent protein kinase. Proc. Natl. Acad. Sci. USA 1991; 88:2011–2015.
35. Nesterova M, Cho-Chung YS. A single-injection protein kinase A-directed antisense treatment to inhibit humor growth. Nat Med 1995; 1:528–633.
36. Agrawal S, Zhao Q. Mixed backbone oligonucleotides: improvement in oligonucleotide-induced toxicity in vivo. Antisense & Nucleic Acid Drug Dev 1998; 8:135–139.
37. Krieg AM, Yi AK, Matson S, et al. CpG motifs in bacterial DNA trigger direct B-cell activation. Nature 1995; 374:546–549.
38. Nesterova M, Cho-Chung YS. Oligonucleotide sequence-specific inhibition of gene expression, tumor growth inhibition, and modulation of cAMP signaling by an RNA-DNA hybrid antisense targeted to protein kinase A RIα subunit. Antisense & Nucleic Acid Drug Development 2000; 10:423–433.
39. Metelev V, Liszlewicz J, Agrawal S. Study of antisense oligonucleotide phosphorothioates containing segments of oligodeoxynucleotides and 2'-O-methyloligoribonucleotides. Bioorg Medicinal Chem Lett 1994; 4:2929–2934.
40. Monia BP, Lesnik EA, Gonzalez C, et al. Evaluation of 2'-modified oligonucleotides containing 2'-deoxygaps as antisense inhibitors of gene expression. J Biol Chem 1993; 268:14514–14522.
41. Shibahara S, Mukai S, Morisawa H, Nakashima H, Kobayashi S, Yamamoto N. Inhibition of human immunodeficiency virus (HIV-1) replication by synthetic oligo-RNA derivatives. Nucleic Acids Res 1989; 17:239–252.
42. Alper O, Hacker NF, Cho-Chung YS. Protein kinase A-Ialpha subunit-directed antisense inhibition of ovarian cancer cell growth: crosstalk with tyrosine kinase signaling pathway. Oncogene 1999; 18:4999–5004.
43. Cho YS, Kim M-K, Tan L, Srivastava R, Agrawal S, Cho-Chung YS. Protein kinase A RIα antisense inhibition of prostate cancer growth: Bcl-2 Hyperphosphorylation, Bax Upregulation, and Bad-Hypophosphorylaton. Clin Cancer Res 2002; 8:607–614.
44. Cho-Chung YS, Nesterova M, Kondrashin A, Noguchi K, Srivastava RK, Pepe S. Antisense-protein kinase A: a single-gene-based therapeutic approach. Antisense & Nucleic Acid Drug Dev 1997; 7:217–223.

45. Nesterova M, Noguchi K, Park YG, Lee YN, Cho-Chung YS. Compensatory stabilization of RIIβ protein, cell cycle deregulation, and growth arrest in colon and prostate carcinoma cells by antisense-directed down-regulation of protein kinase A RIα protein. Clinical Cancer Research 2000; 6:3434–3441.
46. Srivastava RK, Srivastava AR, Seth P, Agrawal S, Cho-Chung YS. Growth arrest and induction of apoptosis in breast cancer cells by antisense depletion of protein kinase A-RI alpha subunit: p53- independent mechanism of action. Mol Cell Biochem 1999; 195:25–36.
47. Srivastava RK, Srivastava AR, Park YG, Agrawal S, Cho-Chung YS. Antisense depletion of RIalpha subunit of protein kinase A induces apoptosis and growth arrest in human breast cancer cells. Breast Cancer Res Treat 1998; 49:97–107.
48. Tortora G, Bianco R, Damiano V, et al. Oral antisense that targets protein kinase A cooperates with taxol and inhibits tumor growth, angiogenesis, and growth factor production. Clin Cancer Res 2000; 6:2506–2512.
49. Wang H, Cai Q, Zeng X, Yu D, Agrawal S, Zhang MQ. Antitumor activity and pharmacokenetics of a mixed-backbone antisense oligonucleotide targeted to the RIα subunit of protein kinase A after oral administration. Proc Natl Acad Sci USA 1999; 96:13989–13994.
50. Amieux PS, Cummings DE, Motamed K, et al. Compensatory regulation of RIalpha protein levels in protein kinase A mutant mice. J Biol Chem 1997; 272:3993–3998.
51. Beavo JA, Reifsnyder DH. Primary sequence of cyclic nucleotide phosphodiesterase isozymes and the design of selective inhibitors. Trends Pharmacol Sci 1990; 11:150–155.
52. Conti M, Jin SL, Monaco L, Repaske DR, Swinnen JV. Hormonal regulation of cyclic nucleotide phosphodiesterases. Endocr Rev 1991; 12:218–234.
53. Neary CL, Cho-Chung YS. Nuclear translocation of the catalytic subunit of protein kinase A induced by an antisense oligonucleotide directed against the RIalpha regulatory subunit. Oncogene 2001; 20:8019–8024.
54. Nesterova M, Cho-Chung YS. Unpublished.
55. Steinberg RA, Agard DA. Turnover of regulatory subunit of cyclic AMP-dependent protein kinase in S49 mouse lymphoma cells. Regulation by catalytic subunit and analogs of cyclic AMP. J Biol Chem 1981; 256:10731–10734.
56. Montminy MR, Bilezikjian LM. Binding of a nuclear protein to the cyclic-AMP response element of the somatostatin gene. Nature 1987; 328:175–178.
57. Gonzalez GA, Biggs W, III, Vale WW, Montminy MR. A cluster of phosphorylation sites on the cyclic AMP-regulated nuclear factor CREB predicated by its sequence. Nature 1989; 337:749–752.
58. Ginty DD, Bonni A, Greenberg ME. Nerve growth factor activates a *ras*-dependent protein kinase that stimulates c-fos transcription via phosphorylation of CREB. Cell 1994; 77:713–725.
59. Rohlff C, Glazer RI. Regulation of multidrug resistance through the cAMP and EGF signaling pathways. Cell Signal 1995; 7:431–443.
60. Chen HX, Marshall JL, Ness E, et al. A safety and pharmacokinetic study of a mixed-backbone oligonucleotide (GEM 231) targeting the type I protein kinase A by 2-hour infusions in patients with refractory solid tumors. Clin Cancer Res 2000; 6:1259–1266.
61. Tortora G, Clair T, Cho-Chung YS. An antisense oligodeoxynucleotide targeted against the type RIIβ regulatory subunit mRNA of protein kinase inhibits cAMP-induced differentiation in HL-60 leukemia cells without affecting phorbol ester effects. Proc Natl Acad Sci USA 1990; 87:705–708.
62. Cho-Chung YS, Clair T, Tortora G, Yokozaki H. Role of site-selective cAMP analogs in the control and reversal of malignancy. Pharmac Ther 1991; 50:1–33.
63. Tortora G, Budillon A, Yokozaki H, et al. Retroviral vector-mediated overexpression of the RIIβ subunit of the cAMP-dependent protein kinase induces differentiation in human leukemia cells and reverts the transformed phenotype of mouse fibroblasts. Cell Growth Differ 1994; 5:753–9.

64. Tortora G, Cho-Chung YS. Type II regulatory subunit of protein kinase restores cAMP-dependent transcription in a cAMP-unresponsive cell line. J Biol Chem 1990; 265:18067–18070.
65. Srivastava RK, Lee YN, Noguchi K, et al. The RIIβ regulatory subunit of protein kinase A binds to cAMP response element: an alternative cAMP signaling pathway. Proc Natl Acad Sci USA 1998; 95:6687–6692.
66. Budillon A, Cereseto A, Kondrashin A, et al. Point mutation of the autophosphorylation site or in the nuclear location signal causes protein kinase A RIIb regulatory subunit to lose its ability to revert transformed fibroblasts. Proc Natl Acad Sci USA 1995; 92:10634–10638.
67. Lohmann SM, Walter U. Regulation of the cellular and subcellular concentrations and distribution of cyclic nucleotide-dependent protein kinases. In: Greengard P, Robinson GA, eds., Advances in cyclic nucleotide and protein phosphorylation research. Vol. 18. New York: Raven Press, 1984:63–117.
68. Cho-Chung YS. Role of cyclic AMP receptor proteins in growth, differentiation, and suppression of malignancy: new approaches to therapy. Cancer Res 1990; 50:7093–7100.
69. Fossberg TM, Døskeland SO, Ueland PM. Protein kinases in human renal cell carcinoma and renal cortex. A comparison of isozyme distribution and of responsiveness to adenosine 3':5'-cyclic monophosphate. Arch Biochem Biophys 1978; 189:272–281.
70. Nakajima F, Imashuku S, Wilimas J, Champion JE, Green AA. Distribution and properties of type I and type II binding proteins in the cyclic adenosine 3':5'-monophosphate-dependent protein kinase system in Wilms' tumor. Cancer Res 1984; 44:5182–5187.
71. Piroli G, Weisenberg LS, Grillo C, De Nicola AF. Subcellular distribution of cyclic adenosine 3',5'-monophosphate- binding protein and estrogen receptors in control pituitaries and estrogen-induced pituitary tumors. J Natl Cancer Inst 1990; 82:596–601.
72. Ekanger R, Øgreid D, Evjen O, Vintermyr O, Laerum OD, Doskeland SO. Characterization of cyclic adenosine 3':5'-monophosphate-dependent protein kinase isozymes in normal and neoplastic fetal rat brain cells. Cancer Res 1985; 45:2578–2583.
73. Livesey SA, Kemp BE, Re CA, Partridge NC, Martin TJ. Selective hormonal activation of cyclic AMP-dependent protein kinase isoenzymes in normal and malignant osteoblasts. J Biol Chem 1982; 257:14983–14987.
74. Schena M, Shalon D, Davis RW, Brown PO. Quantitative monitoring of gene expression patterns with a complementary DNA microarray. Science 1995; 270:467–470.
75. Cho YS, Kim M-K, Cheadle C, Neary C, Becker KG, Cho-Chung YS. Antisense DNAs as multisite genomic modulators identified by DNA microarray. Proc Natl Acad Sci USA 2001; 98:9819–9823.

Index

f: figure
t: table

213

ABOUT THE EDITOR

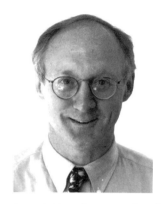

Dr. Gewirtz is a Professor of Medicine and Pathology at the University of Pennsylvania School of Medicine and Leader of the Stem Cell Biology and Therapeutics Program at the University of Pennsylvania Cancer Center. He received his M.D. and M.A. degrees from the State University of New York at Buffalo. Dr. Gewirtz completed his postgraduate training in internal medicine at Mt. Sinai Hospital, New York, and fellowships in Hematology and Oncology at Yale University School of Medicine. Dr. Gewirtz' scientific interests include the cell biology of normal and malignant human hematopoiesis, and translational strategies for silencing gene expression. Dr. Gewirtz was until recently Chair of the Medical and Scientific Affairs Committee of the Leukemia & Lymphoma Society (LLS), and a member of the Experimental Therapeutics-1 NIH Study Section. Presently he serves on the LLS Executive Committee and numerous editorial boards for specialty journals concerned with human stem cells, hematopoiesis, and gene therapy. Dr. Gewirtz has been honored with several awards including the Scientific Achievement Award from the American Cancer Society and the Doris Duke Distinguished Clinical Scientist Award for Excellence in Bench to Bedside Research.